Herpes Simplex Virus Epithelial Keratitis

Helena M. Tabery

Herpes Simplex Virus Epithelial Keratitis

In Vivo Morphology in the Human Cornea

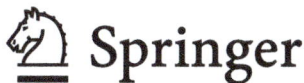
Springer

Helena M. Tabery, MD
Ögonkliniken UMAS
20502 Malmö
Sweden
helena.tabery@telia.com

ISBN: 978-3-642-01011-8   e-ISBN: 978-3-642-01012-5

DOI: 10.1007/978-3-642-01012-5

Springer Heidelberg Dordrecht London New York

Library of Congress Control Number: 2009936007

Cover design: eStudio Calamar, Figueres/Berlin

Printed on acid-free paper

Springer is part of Springer Science+Business Media (www.springer.com)

Preface

As a young ophthalmologist, I found corneal epithelial diseases a subject difficult to grasp. One day, it occurred to me that the reason might be a lack of images showing the nature of the components of the changes visible with the slit lamp. With the slit lamp, the inevitable eye movements that blur the image limited the magnification level, but perhaps photography might be the answer. It was not a short journey, but in the end the idea proved right. By trial and error, the quality of the images improved, and after some time, I found that the resolution allowed reasonable comparisons with available images of histological preparations. Such comparisons allowed better understanding of the substructures of epithelial in vivo lesions and, in conjunction with their in vivo dynamic features, eventually an understanding of at least some mechanisms behind them.

This book, originating from over 20 years of experience with observations of ocular surface changes at high magnification level, covers several aspects of corneal epithelial lesions caused in humans by herpes simplex virus: various shapes of the lesions, their substructure and mechanisms behind them; morphological features of the healing process, sequelae, complications, and some accompanying signs; and some rare cases. For those less familiar with the slit lamp image, I have added explanatory drawings to facilitate comprehension.

It is my experience that once seen at a higher magnification level, these lesions are much easier to recognize with the slit lamp, particularly when the mechanisms behind them are understood. I hope that the reader will discover the same.

Malmö, Sweden
March 2009

Helena M. Tabery

Contents

About Epithelial Keratitis

A healthy corneal epithelium covered by a normally functioning tear film is a prerequisite for the clarity of vision; even minute epithelial changes located in the optical zone impair visual acuity. Epithelial malfunction may also result in serious damage to the subjacent stromal tissue, such as scarring or corneal melting and perforation. The differential diagnosis of epithelial diseases might be easy but also difficult because they often resemble each other. The reason is the paucity of morphological phenomena occurring in the epithelium as a reaction to noxious stimuli, whether external (e.g., various forms of injuries, including virus infections), innate to the individual (e.g., dystrophies and manifestations of diseases such as rosacea and atopy), or of unknown causes (e.g., Thygeson's keratitis). Individual phenomena occurring in these conditions (e.g., cell swelling, cyst formation, diseased surface cells, abnormal cells) are per se not disease specific. It is their combination and distribution, both in depth and laterally, sometimes in conjunction with their dynamic features, that make them relatable to a specific disease.

About Herpes Simplex Virus Epithelial Keratitis

Herpes simplex virus (HSV) corneal epithelial infections are very common. *Primary eye infections*, that is, those caused by virus transmission between individuals, may be subclinical or manifest as a self-limiting conjunctivitis that passes undiagnosed. Primary epithelial keratitis is only rarely seen, or diagnosed, particularly in an adult. After the primary event, the virus is not eliminated from the organism; instead, it travels by retrograde flow to neuron cell bodies in the trigeminal ganglion supplying the eye and remains there in a latent state. The virus that infects the eye might have gained access to the trigeminal ganglion also during facial infections, usually around the mouth. The large majority of HSV epithelial keratitis seen in clinical practice are *recurrences* caused by shedding of reactivated virus. They are usually caused by HSV-1 (type 1); so far, HSV-2 (type 2, genital herpes) is rarely encountered.

Herpes simplex virus can seriously damage the eye. The recognition of the HSV origin of *epithelial keratitis* is of great importance not only to avoid confusion with other conditions but also because it may be a clue to help identify HSV as a cause of a more serious eye involvement, such as stromal keratitis or uveitis. Such manifestations may precede or follow epithelial keratitis, both within a short time frame or many years apart.

Herpes simplex virus epithelial keratitis is largely known as a *branching figure (dendrite)*. To diagnose *nonbranching lesions*, particularly small ones, as herpetic and to differentiate dendritic lesions from other lesions also showing branching patterns (e.g., herpes zoster, Thygeson's keratitis, healing erosions, recurrent erosions), it is mandatory to carefully observe both their shapes and their substructures.

Treatment with antiviral drugs that arrest virus replication (e.g., acyclovir ointment) causes rapid changes in the morphology of epithelial keratitis. Knowledge of the typical *healing pattern* is helpful in differentiating successful treatment from treatment failure, and knowledge of *side effects of treatment* helps differentiate them from epithelial infection.

Successful treatment eradicates replicating virus from the corneal epithelium. The treatment, however early it starts ($\leq$24 h after onset), does not prevent the development of subepithelial damage (often termed *ghost* figure), which in some individuals disappears rapidly but in others clears only slowly and sometimes remains indefinitely. This sequela might be helpful in suspecting a previous herpetic infection; however, it might be indistinguishable from sequelae of other epithelial virus infections, such as adenovirus and herpes zoster.

About This Book

The photographs presented in this book have been chosen to show

– The *in vivo morphology* of herpes simplex virus (HSV) corneal epithelial infection and the mechanisms behind it (Chap. 1)
– The *morphology of healing* of HSV lesions treated with a topical antiviral drug (acyclovir) and the morphology of short-term sequelae of the infection (Chap. 2)
– Five *illustrative cases* with complications, accompanying signs, recurrences, and long-term sequelae of the infection (Chap. 3)

The photographs were taken by *noncontact in vivo photomicrography,* a method that requires neither contact with the epithelium nor the use of anesthetics. By this method, structures that optically differ from their regularly organized surroundings are visualized; a normal corneal epithelium or stromal cells cannot be discerned. As there is no contact with the ocular surface, the architecture of epithelial changes is not disturbed during the examination, and there is no risk of spreading infection in diseases such as HSV. The technique allows the use of various illumination modes to complement each other and a free application of *diagnostic dyes* to expand the information, e.g. 1% fluorescein sodium and 1% rose bengal (preservative-free solutions). These dyes are commonly used in clinical practice.

The photographs of cell cultures were taken by the same method.

The *HSV origin* (type 1) of the lesions was verified by virus isolation test; in two cases, the diagnosis was clinical.

The *bars* indicate *200 µm throughout the book.*

Abbreviations

HSV	Herpes simplex virus
CPE	Cytopathic effect
Fluorescein	Fluorescein sodium

Chapter 1

The Morphology of Herpes Simplex Virus Epithelial Keratitis

Before the introduction of newer methods, the gold standard of detection and identification of viruses was virus isolation test in *cell culture*. In living cells, virus replication causes cell swelling and rounding (a phenomenon termed the *virus cytopathic effect*, CPE) followed by cell bursting and disappearance.

When the multilayered living human *corneal epithelium* in situ becomes infected with HSV, the virus CPE generates *secondary phenomena*: Subsurface cell swelling causes volume increase, resulting in *surface elevations* and *disruptions*; subsequent shedding of surface cells, and bursting and disappearance of infected ones, causes loss of substance, resulting in *surface depressions* (epithelial erosions/ulcerations). This sequence of events often occurs asynchronously. The *early stages* of the infection clearly show a concurrent presence of incipient cell swelling and advanced epithelial destruction; in fact, it is the blended substructure due to the presence in adjacent areas of various degrees of epithelial damage that greatly contributes to the familiar appearance of HSV epithelial lesions.

Among the various shapes of HSV lesions, one occupies an outstanding position: the well-known *herpetic dendrite*. The possible mechanisms behind these branching figures often showing "terminal bulbs" (rounded branch endings) have been debated for many years. Helpful in elucidating this question is the initial distribution of infected cells captured during the very early stages; it indicates that the patterns of the dendrites are laid down early. That the variously shaped figures are the result of confluence of adjacent foci of infection, larger and smaller, is also clearly visible in fresh dendrites.

Lesions that do not show the "HSV-typical" shapes are less common and might be a diagnostic pitfall: small lesions, oval or rounded, singular or multiple, resembling adenovirus infections; lesions with configurations reminiscent of mechanical injuries; elongated lesions lacking "terminal bulbs"; lesions that had lost their original features because of extensive epithelial destruction ("geographic" lesions). In such lesions, HSV features can be easily overlooked unless the examination is careful.

It is well known that HSV epithelial keratitis is a self-limiting condition. Participation of natural defensive forces during ongoing infection seems reflected by the fairly well-defined configurations of lesions in patients presenting several days, or later, after the onset of symptoms; in fact, this phenomenon would be difficult to understand without presupposing a force hindering free lateral spreading of the infection. I can recall only two patients in whom the infection seemed to have progressed unopposed. One was a rare case of primary infection (presented in this chapter); in the other one, swollen/rounded cells scattered over a largely epithelium-denuded corneal surface were reminiscent of advanced changes in cell cultures. This patient had inadvertently been treated with a potent topical steroid.

H. M. Tabery, *Herpes Simplex Virus Epithelial Keratitis*
DOI: 978-3-642-01012-5_1, © Springer-Verlag Berlin Heidelberg 2010

HSV Cytopathic Effect: Early Changes

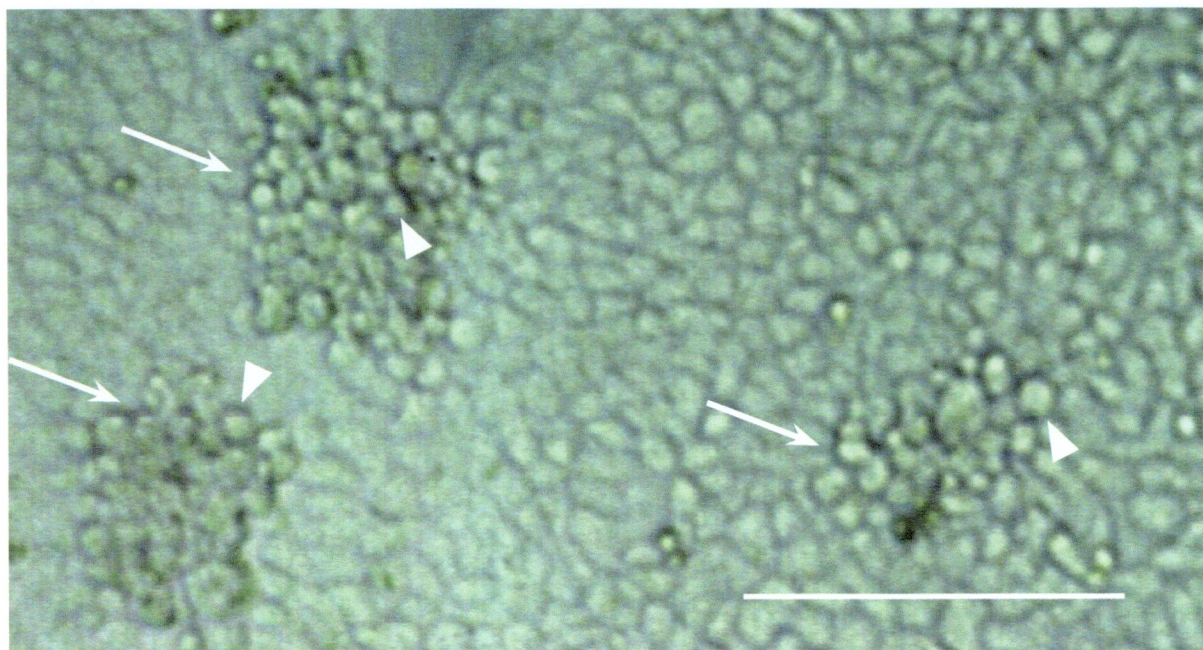

Fig. 1.1 HSV cytopathic effect in *cell culture* infected with a laboratory strain of HSV type 1 (HSV-1). The figure shows foci (*arrows*) containing swollen/rounded infected cells (*arrowheads*)

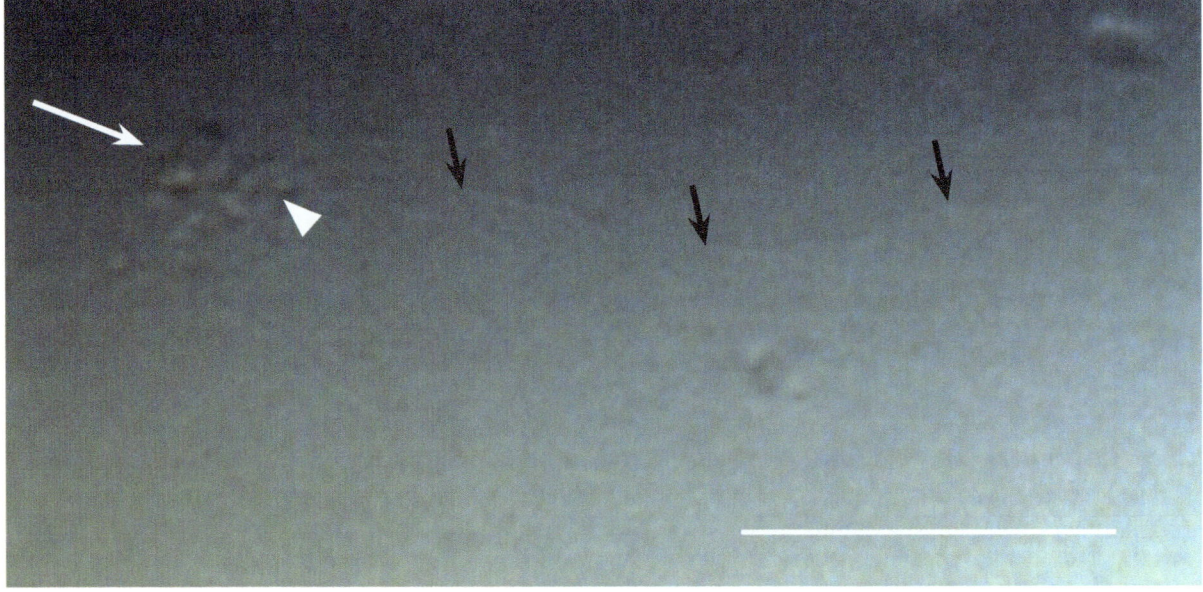

Fig. 1.2 In the *living human corneal epithelium*, incipient HSV cytopathic effect appears as foci (*white arrow*) containing swollen/rounded cells (*arrowhead*). *Black arrows* indicate a corneal nerve

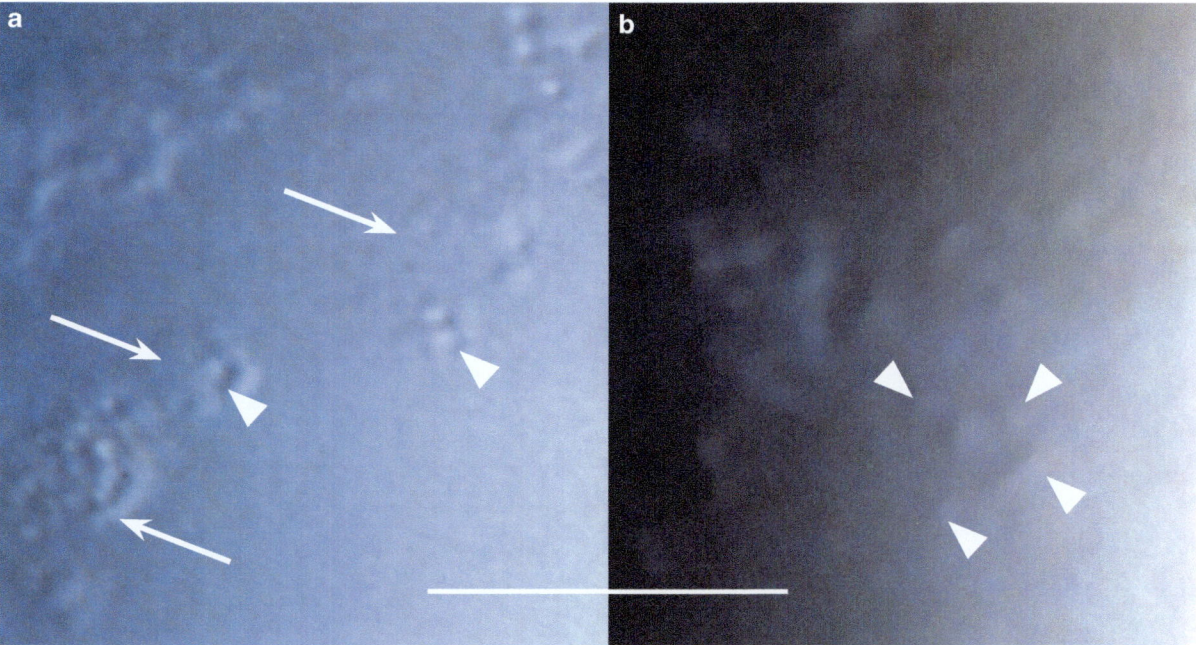

Fig. 1.3 a–b HSV cytopathic effect in the *living human corneal epithelium*. (**a**) Several partly confluent foci (*arrows*) containing swollen/rounded cells (*arrowheads*). (**b**) Individual swollen/rounded cells (*arrowheads*) close to each other

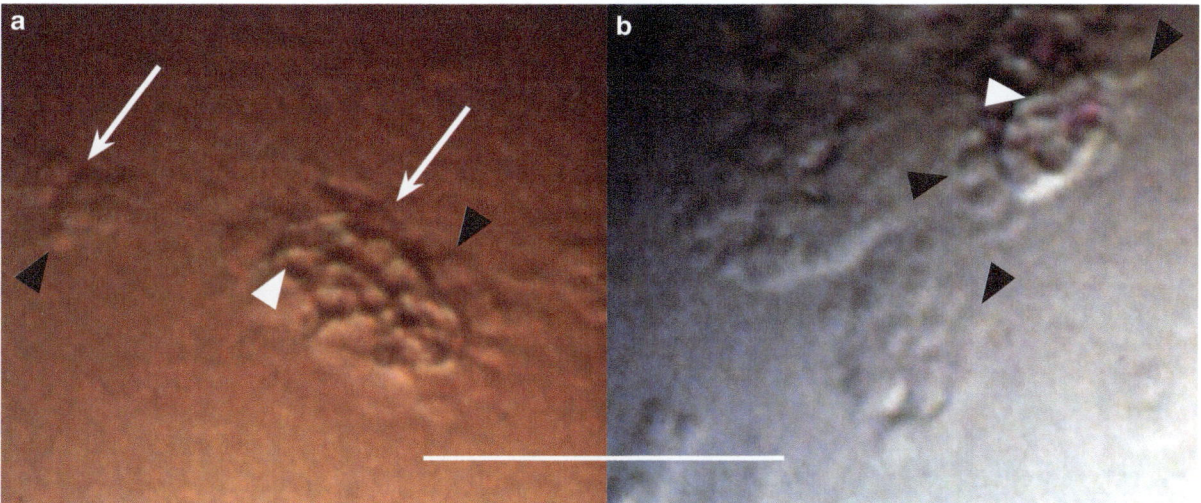

Fig. 1.4 a–b HSV cytopathic effect in the *living human corneal epithelium*. (**a**) Two adjacent foci (*arrows*) containing swollen/ rounded cells (*arrowheads*). In the left focus, and in the periphery of the right one, the cells appear dull (*black arrowheads*). In the center of the right focus are visible bright rounded cells (*white arrowhead*); here, the surface layer seems missing. (**b**) As in (**a**), the dull-appearing cells (*black arrowheads*) seem situated below a preserved surface layer, and the bright ones (*white arrowhead*) appear denuded. A few cells stained red with rose bengal

Comment

The condition of the surface can be visualized with fluorescein sodium (cf. Fig. 1.10).

HSV Cytopathic Effect: Advanced Changes

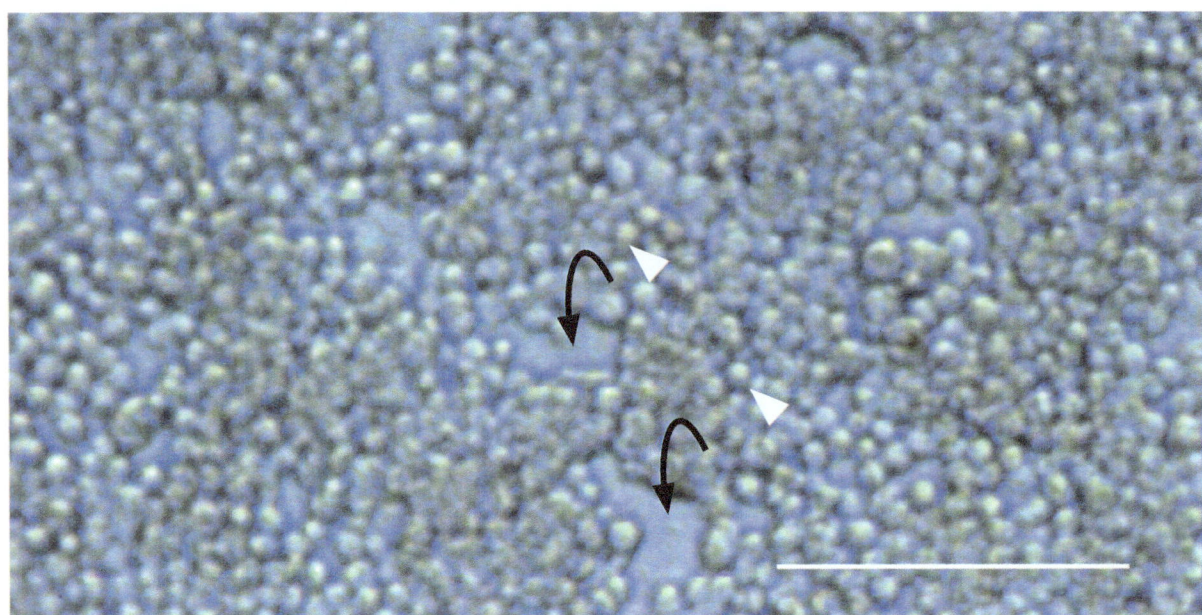

Fig. 1.5 This *cell culture* infected with a laboratory (HSV-1) virus strain shows advanced changes: All remaining cells show the virus cytopathic effect (cell swelling and rounding, *arrowheads*); moreover, in the cell monolayer, cell bursting and disappearance have resulted in cell-denuded areas (*arrows*)

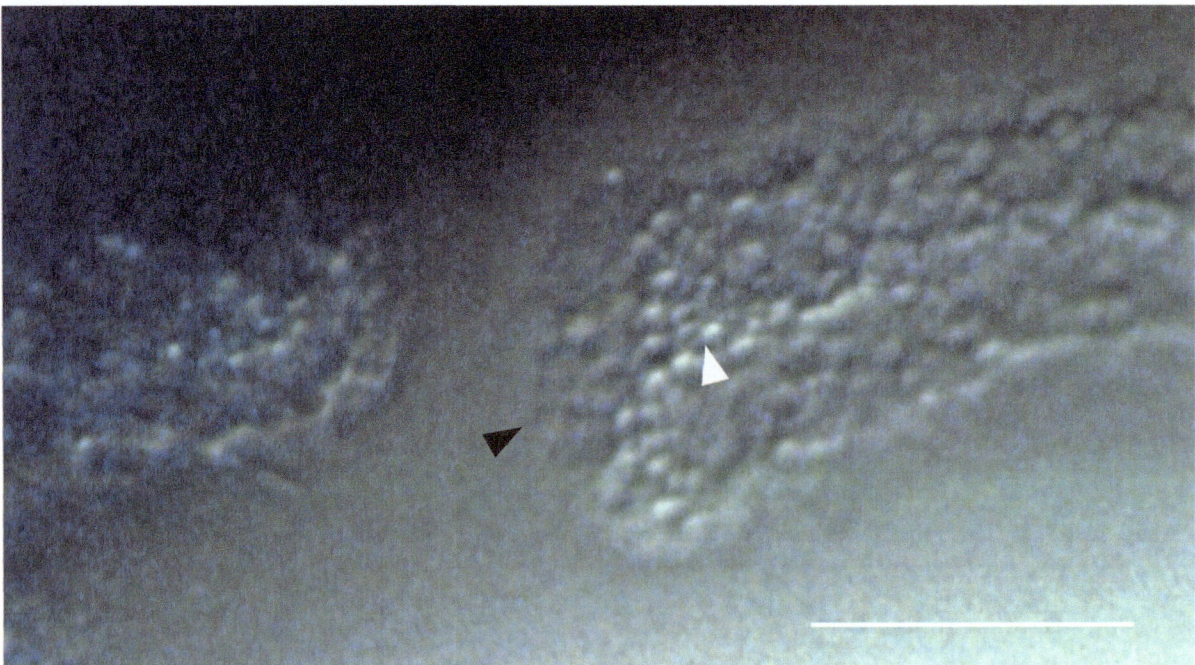

Fig. 1.6 This HSV lesion in the *living human corneal epithelium* shows closely packed swollen/rounded cells, some appearing dull (*black arrowhead*) and others bright (*white arrowhead*); in the multilayered epithelium, cell bursting and disappearance have not resulted in cell-denuded areas yet (cf. Fig. 1.7, opposite page)

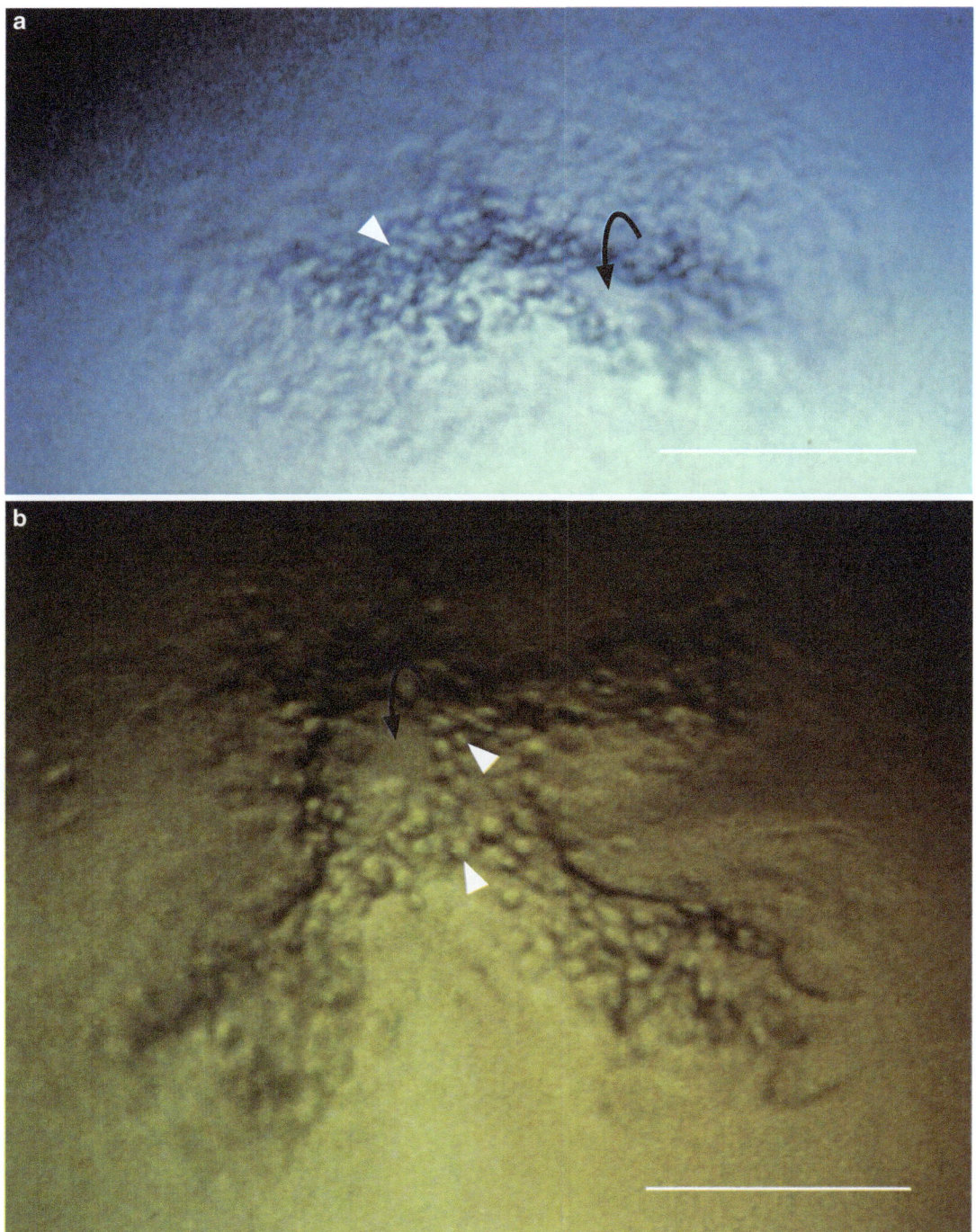

Fig. 1.7 a–b The appearance of these two HSV lesions in the *living human corneal epithelium* is the result of cell swelling (*arrowheads*), bursting, and disappearance. In places, the loss of substance seems to have reached the level of the epithelial basement membrane (*arrows* indicate apparently cell-denuded areas)

Level differences can be visualized with fluorescein sodium (cf. Fig.1.9).

Early HSV In Vivo Lesions: Surface Elevation and Disruption

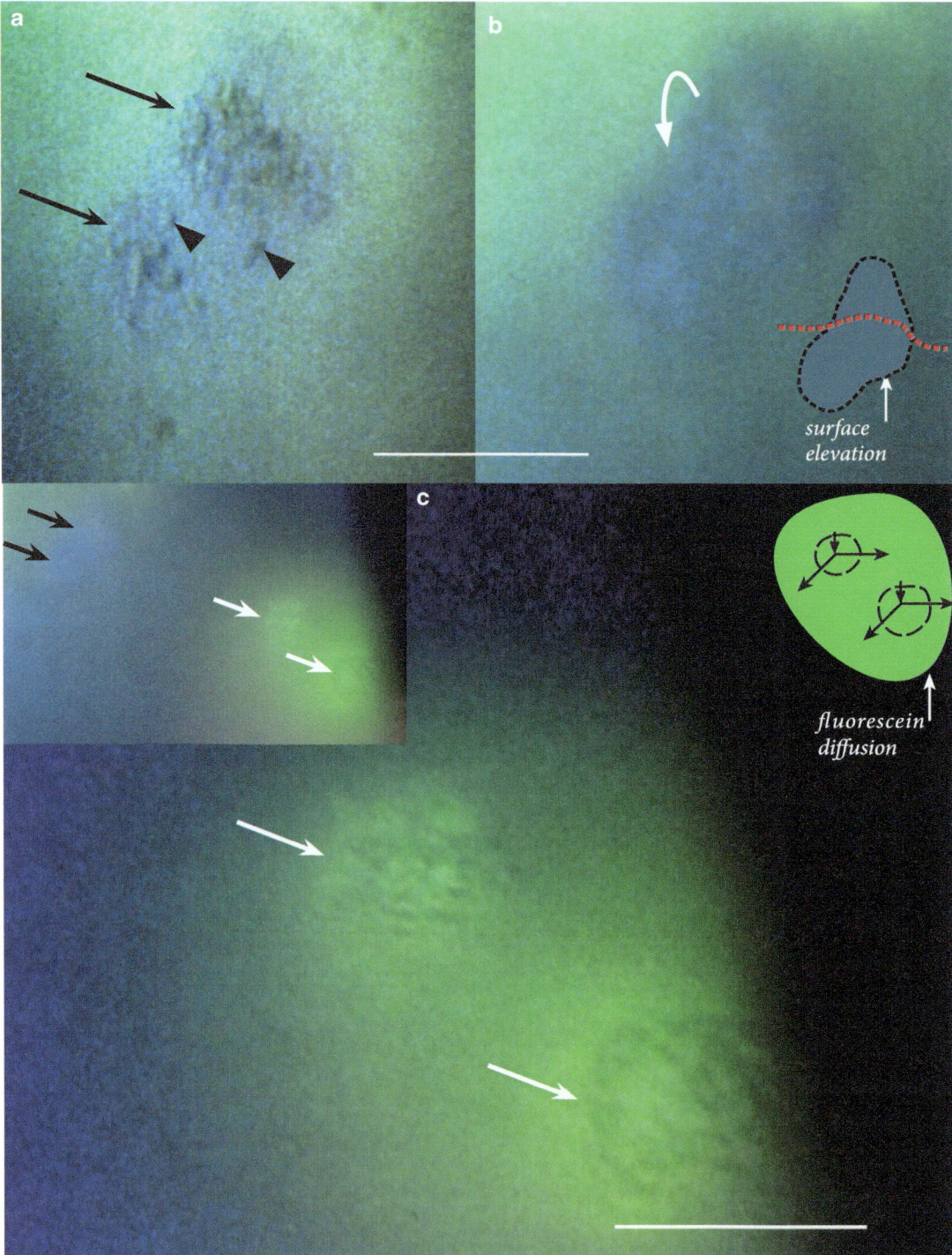

Fig. 1.8 a–c (**a**) In these two confluent HSV epithelial lesions (*arrows*), cell swelling (*arrowheads*) causes (**b**) surface elevation (dark in the tear film stained green with fluorescein sodium, *arrow*). The surface layer is preserved (no diffusion). (**c**) Two other lesions (*arrows*) show massive diffusion of fluorescein, indicating loss of surface integrity. *Inset:* Both types of lesions are located close to each other

An Advanced HSV In Vivo Lesion: Loss of Substance

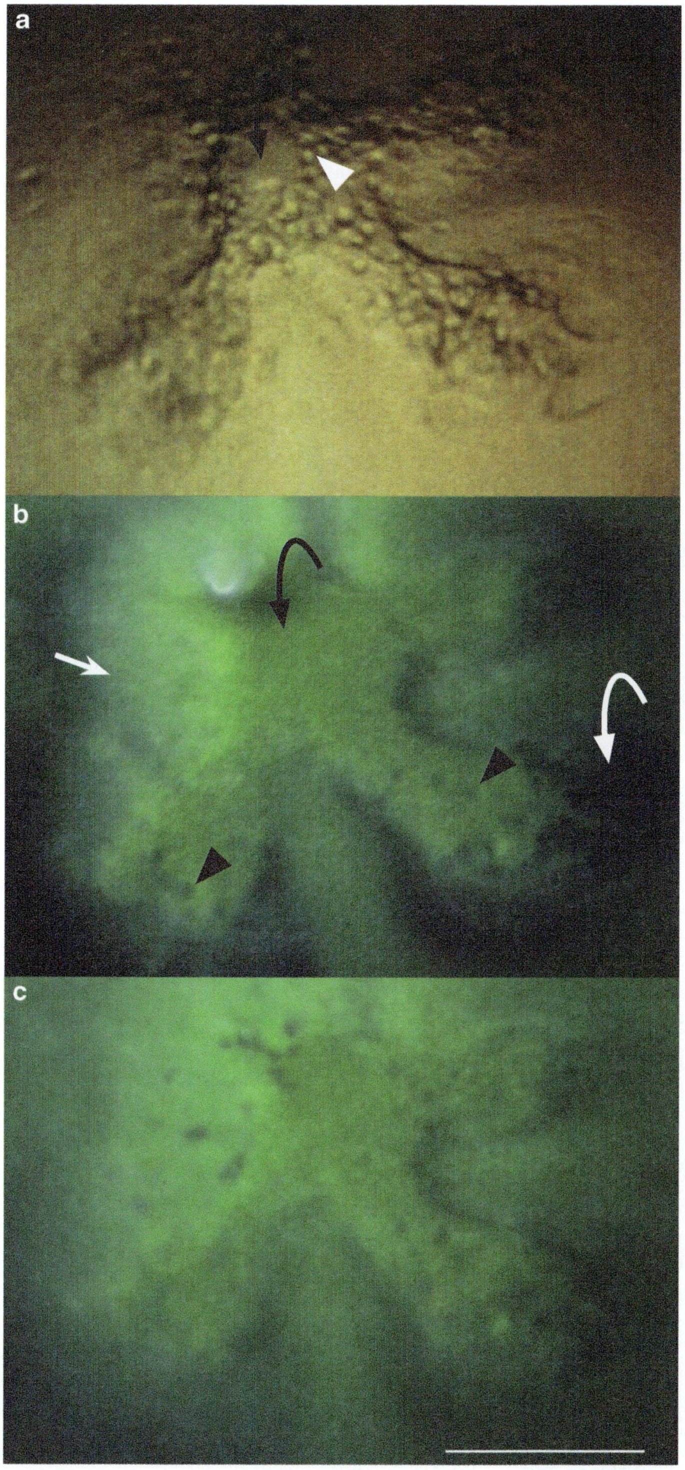

(**a**) Loss of substance caused by epithelial destruction resulted in surface erosion (depression). The bottom of the lesion shows swollen/rounded cells (*arrowhead*) and a partly cell-denuded area (*arrow*)

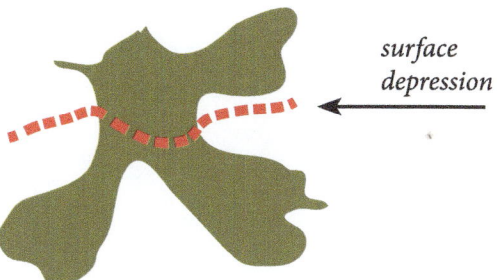

(**b**) The eroded (depressed) area (*bowed black arrow*) shows pooling of green-stained tear fluid. The majority of the swollen cells visible in (**a**) have disappeared below the level of the fluid; only a few cells are protruding (*arrowheads*). Elevated areas adjacent to the depressed ones appear dark (*bowed white arrow*); early fluorescein diffusion into the surroundings appears bright green (*short arrow*)

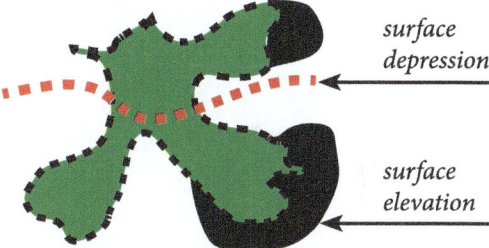

(**c**) The bright green fluorescein staining caused by diffusion into the surroundings increases with time

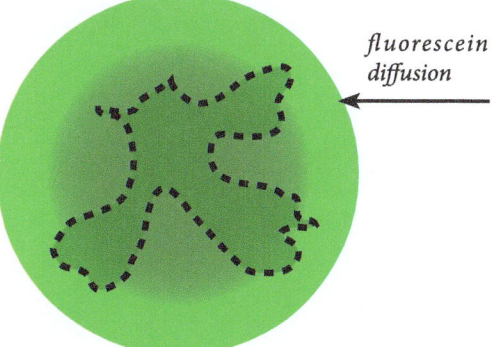

Fig. 1.9 a–c A part of an advanced HSV dendrite before and after the application of fluorescein sodium. (Adapted from [2])

HSV Lesions: Surface Elevation, Depression, and Fluid Diffusion

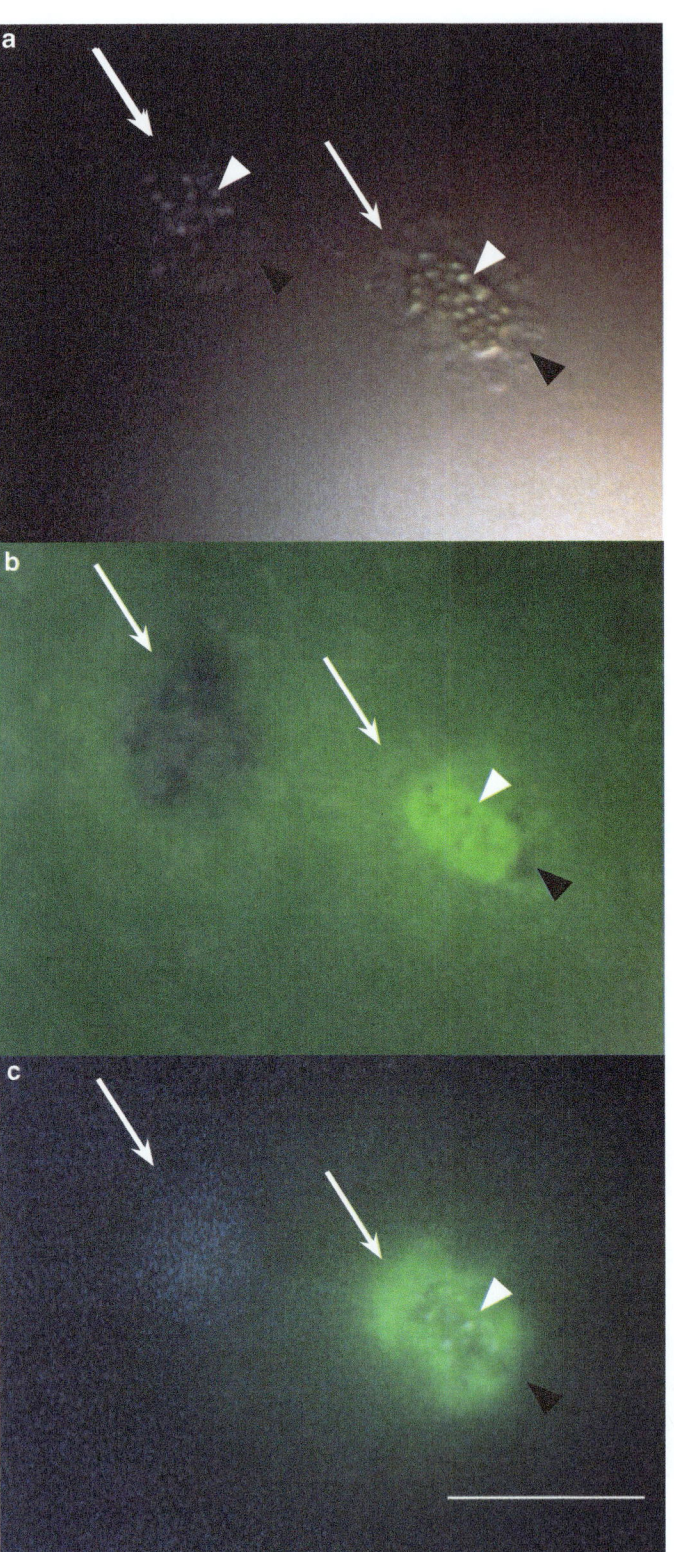

Fig. 1.10 a–c The same area visualized without and with fluorescein sodium. The markers are placed in corresponding locations. (Adapted from [5])

(**a**) Before the application of the dye, two small foci are visible (*arrows*). Both show "bright" (*white arrowheads*) and "dull" (*black arrowheads*) swollen/rounded cells. The center of the right focus seems depressed

(**b**) Tear fluid stained green with fluorescein sodium discloses that the surface of the left focus is partly elevated (dark). In the right focus, the dye is pooling within a surface depression (missing substance). Some swollen/rounded cells are discernible within the depression (*white arrowhead*); others are slightly protruding at the edge (*black arrowhead*)

(**c**) After a couple of minutes, the dye has disappeared from the tear film. The left focus appears grayish; no fluorescein diffusion has occurred. The right focus shows fluorescein diffusion into the area surrounding the depression (*black arrowhead*) and into the surroundings of the lesion

(The healing of these two lesions is shown in Fig. 2.1).

HSV Lesions: Epithelial and Stromal Fluid Diffusion

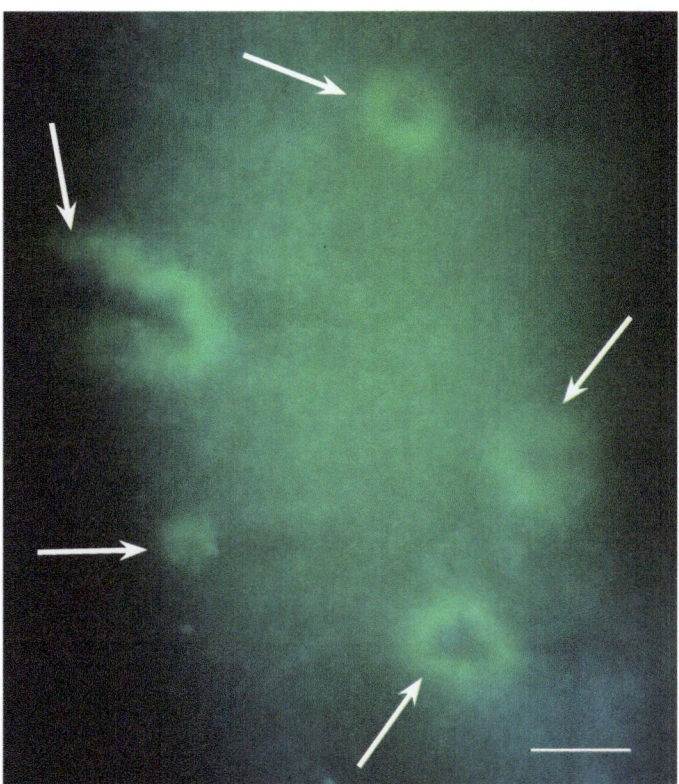

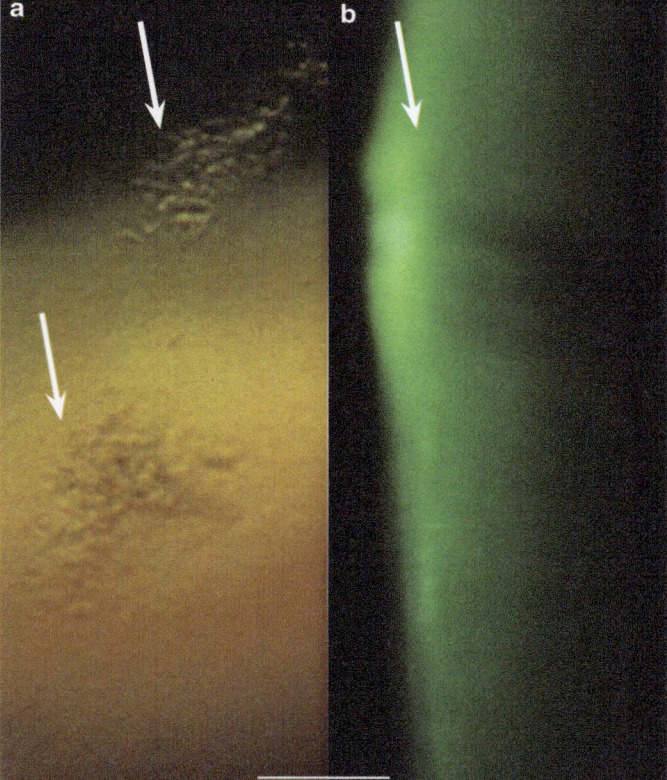

Fig. 1.11 a–b Small HSV lesions (*arrows*) close to each other. Fluorescein sodium has disappeared from the tear film. Fluorescein diffusion into the epithelium appears as bright green halos surrounding disrupted, or eroded, areas. In addition, the whole area between them is stained green. Whether such diffusion occurs within the epithelium only or also concerns the subepithelial tissues cannot be judged in a two-dimensional photograph; however, it can be detected in optical section of the cornea (cf. Fig. 1.12)

Optical Section Through the Cornea

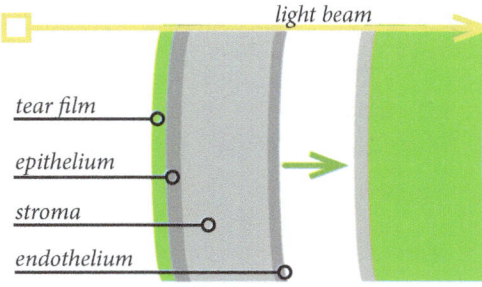

Left: Tear film overlying the corneal epithelium is stained green with fluorescein sodium
Right: Fluorescein sodium has penetrated through surface disruptions into the epithelium and the underlying stroma; the dye has disappeared from the tear film

Fig. 1.12 a–b (**a**) Two small HSV lesions (*arrows*) close to each other. (**b**) Optical section through the corneal epithelium and stroma in the area of the upper lesion shown in (**a**, *arrow*). By diffusion of fluorescein sodium, the epithelium and the stroma stain green

Rose Bengal Dye Staining of HSV Lesions

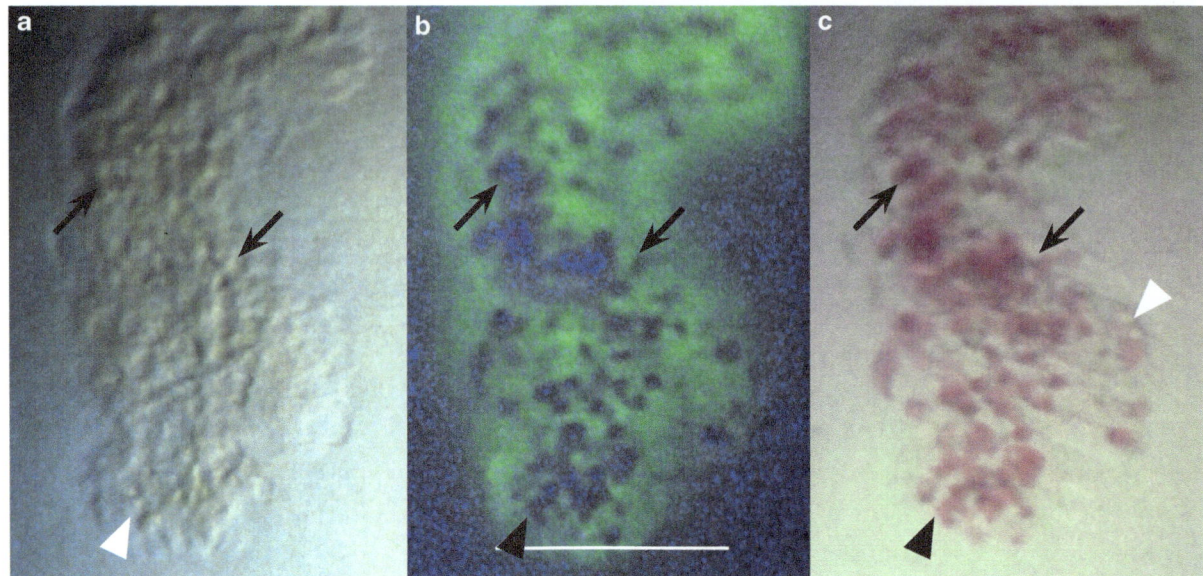

Fig. 1.13 a–c Lower part of a large HSV lesion. *Arrows* indicate corresponding locations. (**a**) Before staining, the lesion shows many closely packed swollen/rounded cells (*arrowhead*). (**b**) With fluorescein sodium, the lesion stains green. Diseased/damaged surface cells stained with rose bengal appear as dark red-bluish dots (*arrowhead*). In places, the staining is confluent. (**c**) Some swollen/rounded cells stain red with rose bengal (*black arrowhead*); others do not (*white arrowhead*)

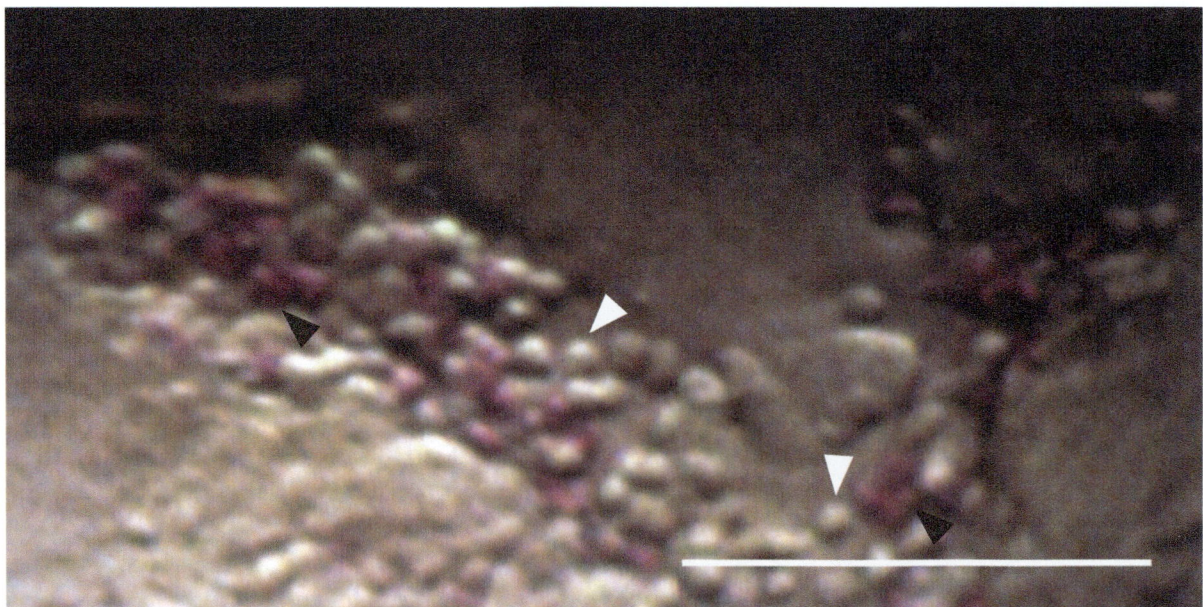

Fig. 1.14 Part of an HSV lesion showing many swollen/rounded cells. Some stain with rose bengal (*black arrowheads*); others do not (*white arrowheads*)

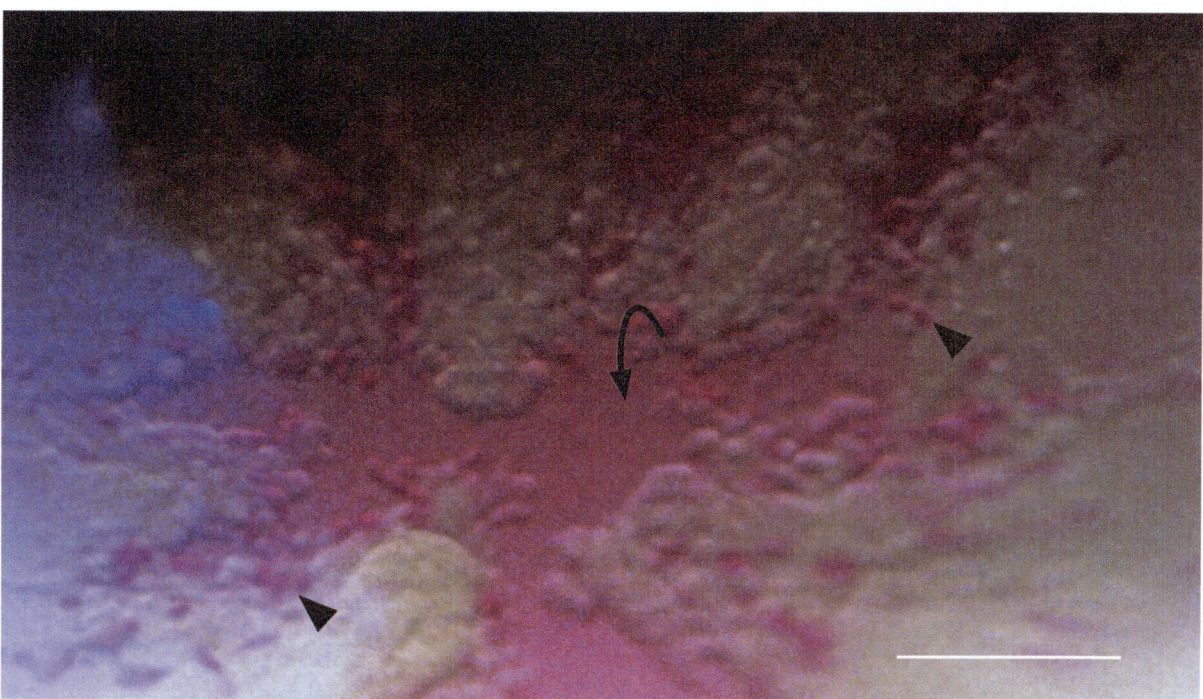

Fig. 1.15 In this erosive (dendrogeographic) HSV lesion, the cell-denuded bottom (*arrow*) stains red with rose bengal. Some swollen/rounded cells also stain red with the dye (*arrowheads*). (Adapted from [7])

Comment

Which of the swollen/rounded cells are virus infected and which represent an unspecific phenomenon cannot be decided (additional features of this lesion are shown in Chap. 3, Case 1)

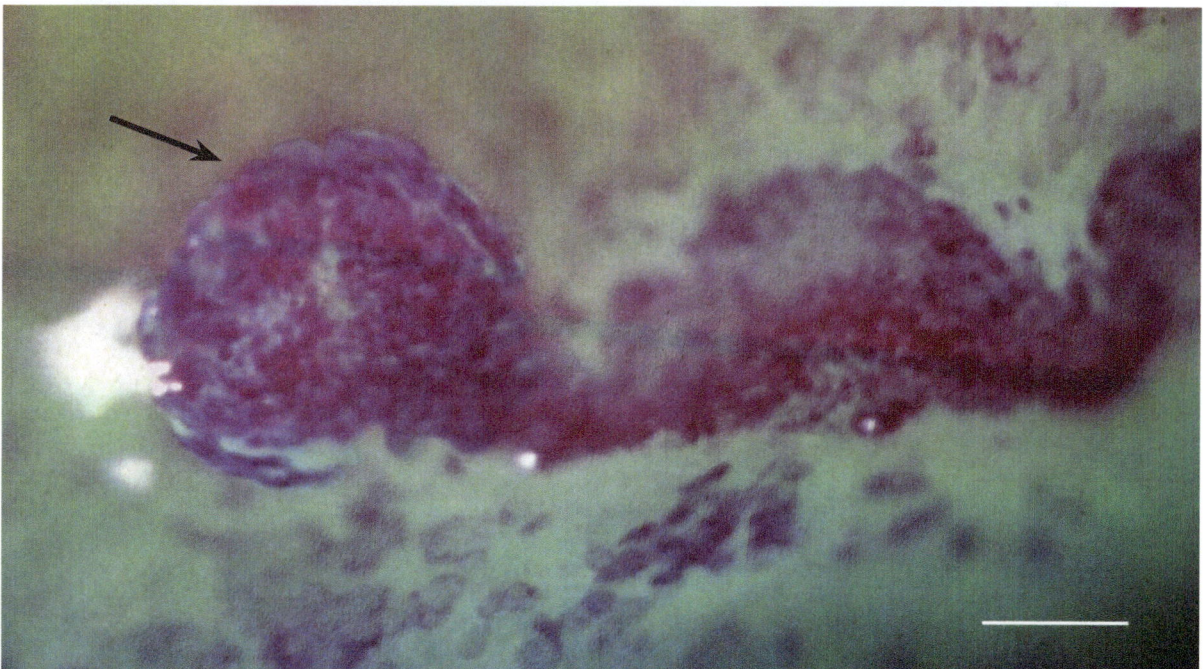

Fig. 1.16 In this cornea, the epithelium was edematous over the whole surface. In one location, an epithelial lesion was suspected but difficult to discern. The whole epithelium stained rapidly with fluorescein sodium. Rose bengal dye revealed a lesion (*arrow*) suggestive of an HSV infection

An HSV Dendritic Figure

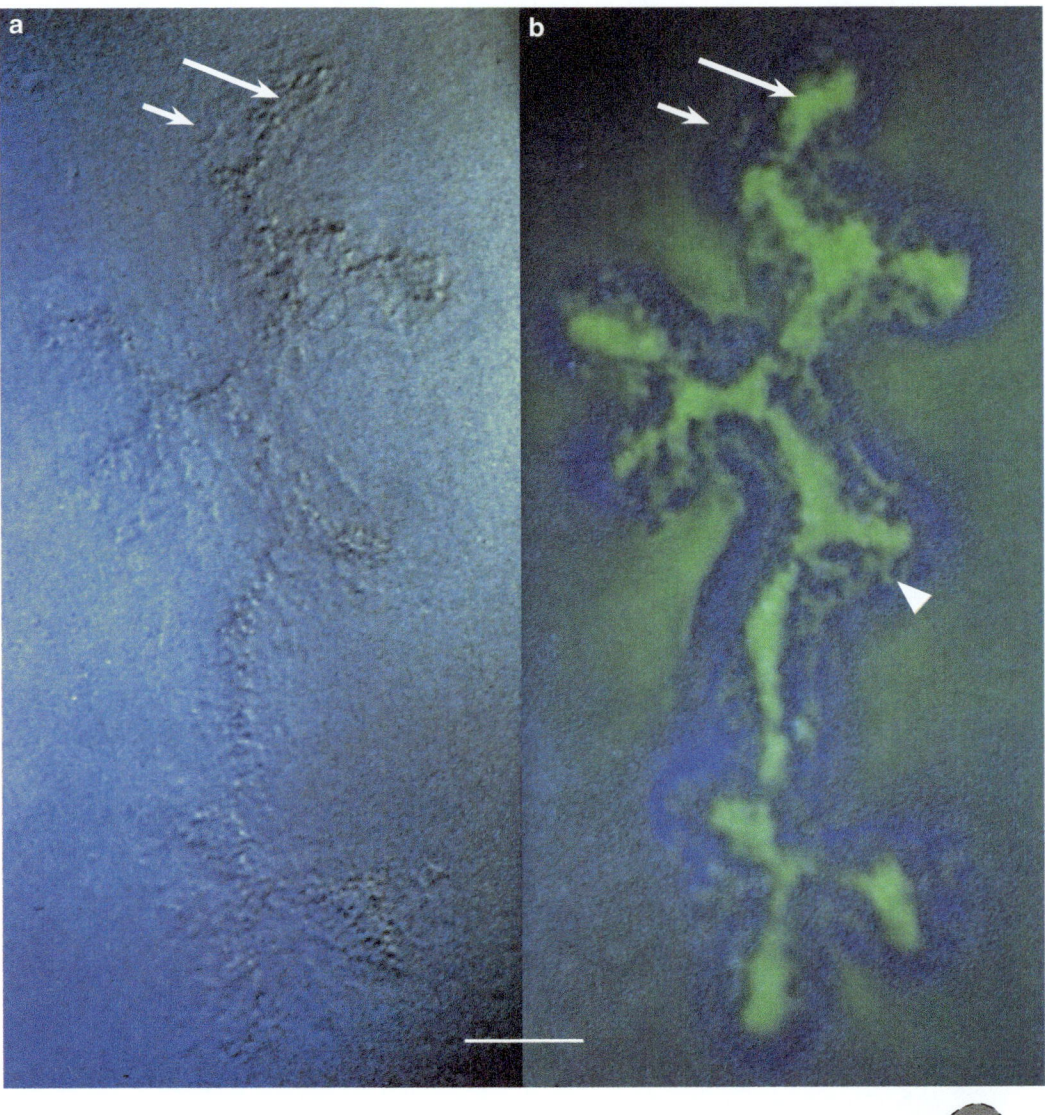

Fig. 1.17 a–d Features of an HSV dendritic (branching) figure, visualized (**a**) without staining, (**b** and **c**) with fluorescein sodium, (**c** and **d**) in time sequence, and (**d**) with rose bengal dye added. (**a**) The figure consist of two parts: a central core that appears granular (*long arrow*) and a surrounding zone (*short arrow*) (cf. drawing). (**b**) Green-stained tear fluid is pooling within the central core. The surrounding zone is elevated (dark). Within this zone, green fluid is pooling between protruding swollen/rounded cells (dark rounded dots, *arrowhead*)

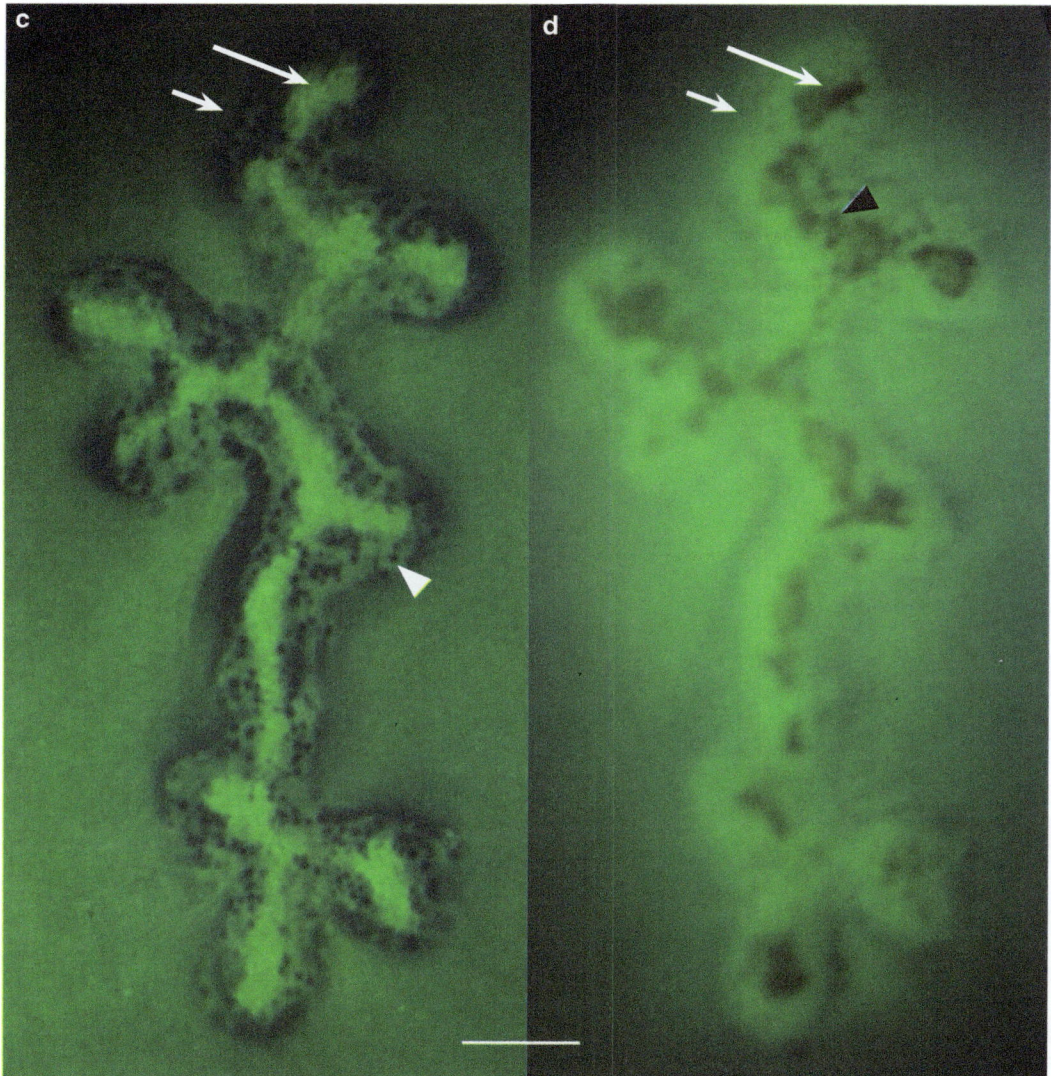

Fig. 1.17 (c) After a blink, the stained tear fluid appears more brilliantly green. As in (**b**), it is pooling within the central core and between the protruding swollen/rounded cells (*arrowhead*). So far, there is no fluorescein diffusion into the elevated surrounding zone. (**d**) A few minutes later, the elevated surrounding zone is stained brilliantly green (fluorescein diffusion). Rose bengal dye reveals patches of surface debris within the central core and a few rounded dots (*arrowhead*)

Comment

*It is possible that the pooling of the green-stained tear fluid captured within the central core in (**b**) and (**c**) occurs below a damaged but partially preserved surface layer.*

An HSV Dendritic Figure (Continued)

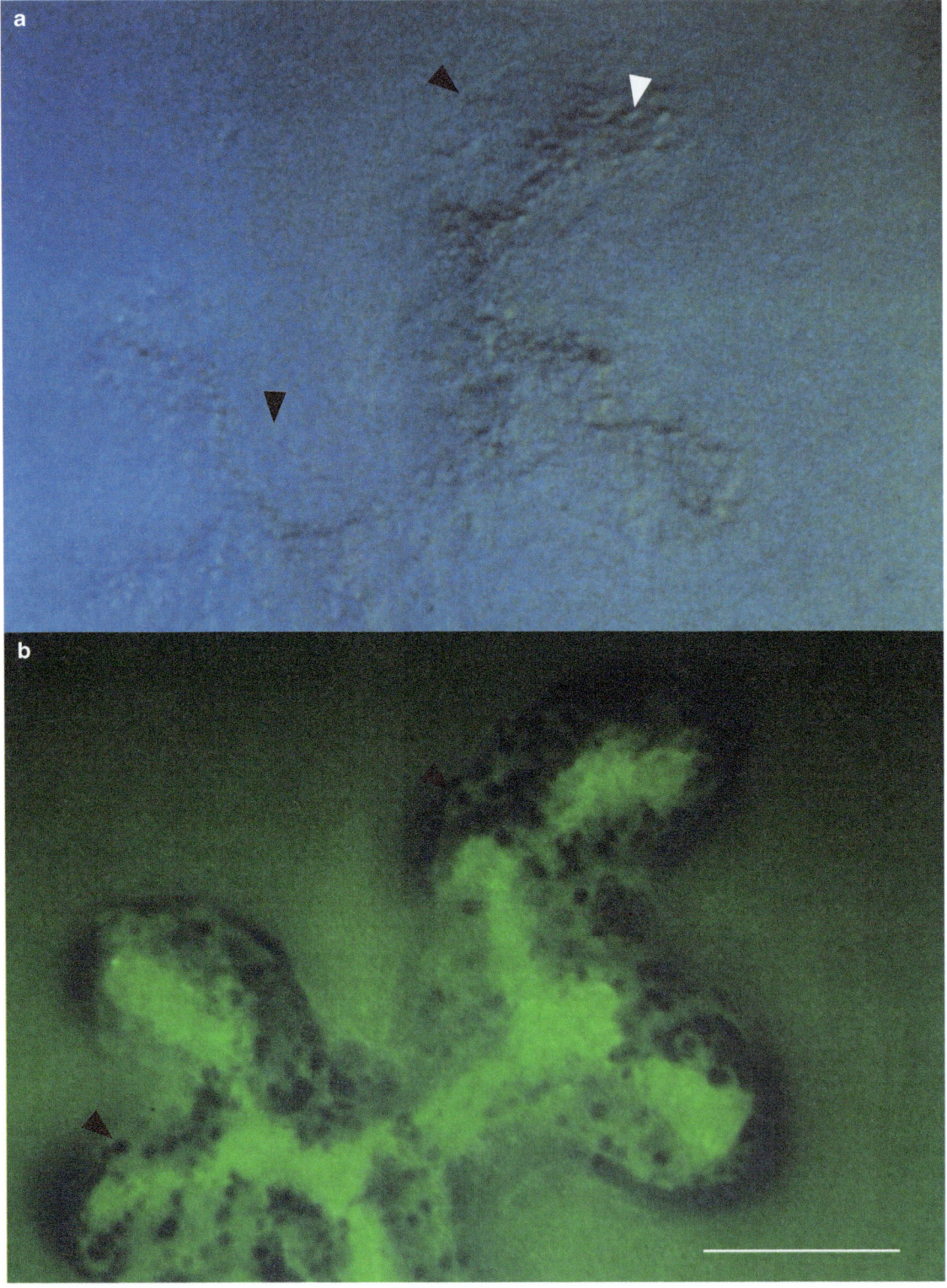

Fig. 1.18 a–b Close view of the upper part of the dendrite shown in Fig. 1.17. (**a**) Swollen/rounded cells within the central core (*white arrowhead*) and in the surrounding zone (*black arrowheads*). (**b**) Protruding swollen/rounded cells appear as dark rounded dots (*black arrowheads*) surrounded by green-stained fluid

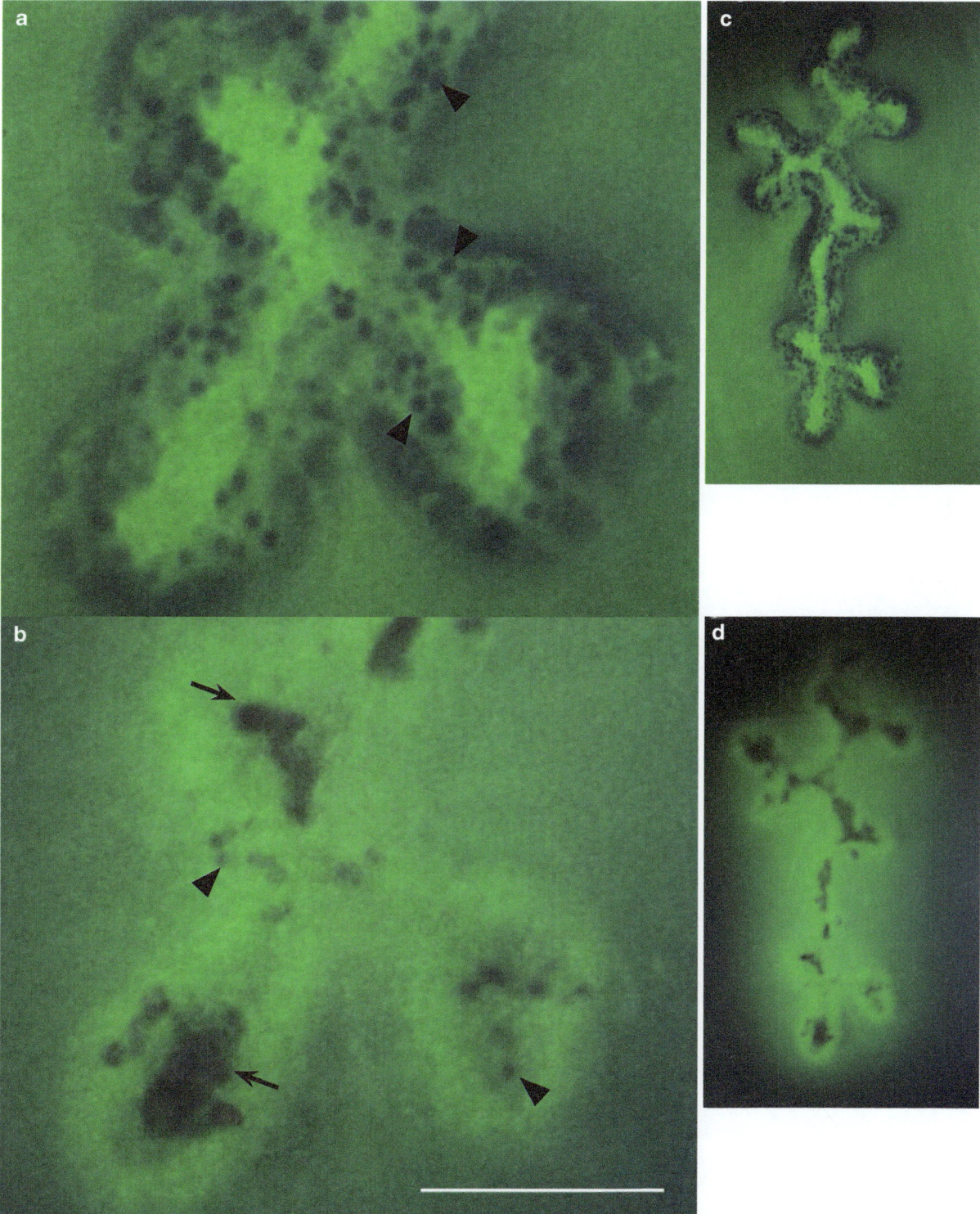

Fig. 1.19 **a–d** Close view of the lower part of the dendrite shown in Fig. 1.17. (**a**) The surrounding zone shows many protruding swollen cells (*arrowheads*). (**b**) The surrounding zone stains brilliantly green (fluorescein diffusion). Cell debris (*arrows*) and a few diseased cells (*arrowheads*) stain red with rose bengal. (**c–d**) Survey of the same figure. (**c**) Green-stained tear fluid reveals elevated edges (*dark*) of the dendrite and fluid pooling within the dendrite. (**d**) Fluorescein diffusion into the epithelium within and outside the dendrite successively transforms the whole area into a green fleck in which morphological details are difficult or impossible to discern

The Origin of HSV Dendritic Figures

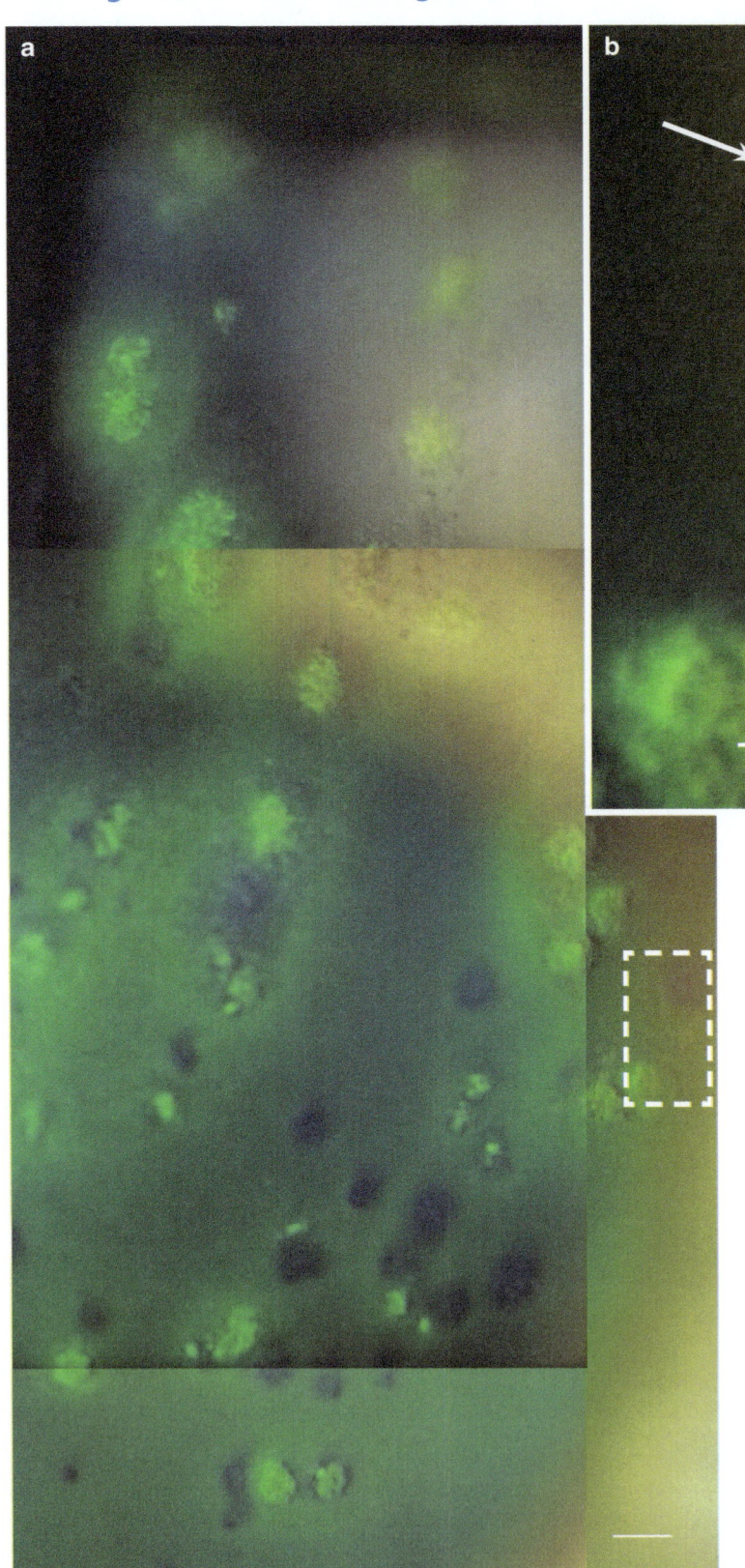

Fig. 1.20 a–b (**a**) This cornea, captured within 24 h after onset of symptoms, shows many small HSV lesions spread over the surface (composed photograph). The various shapes of HSV figures (Fig. 1.21), branching or not, are the result of random confluence of smaller and larger lesions. (**b**) Close view of the area indicated by frame in (**a**); the confluence of individual foci is clearly visible. The upper lesion (*arrow*) might be a precursor of a terminal bulb (i.e., a rounded enlargement often seen at branch endings, cf. Fig. 1.23). (Adapted from [5])

Various Shapes of HSV Dendritic Figures

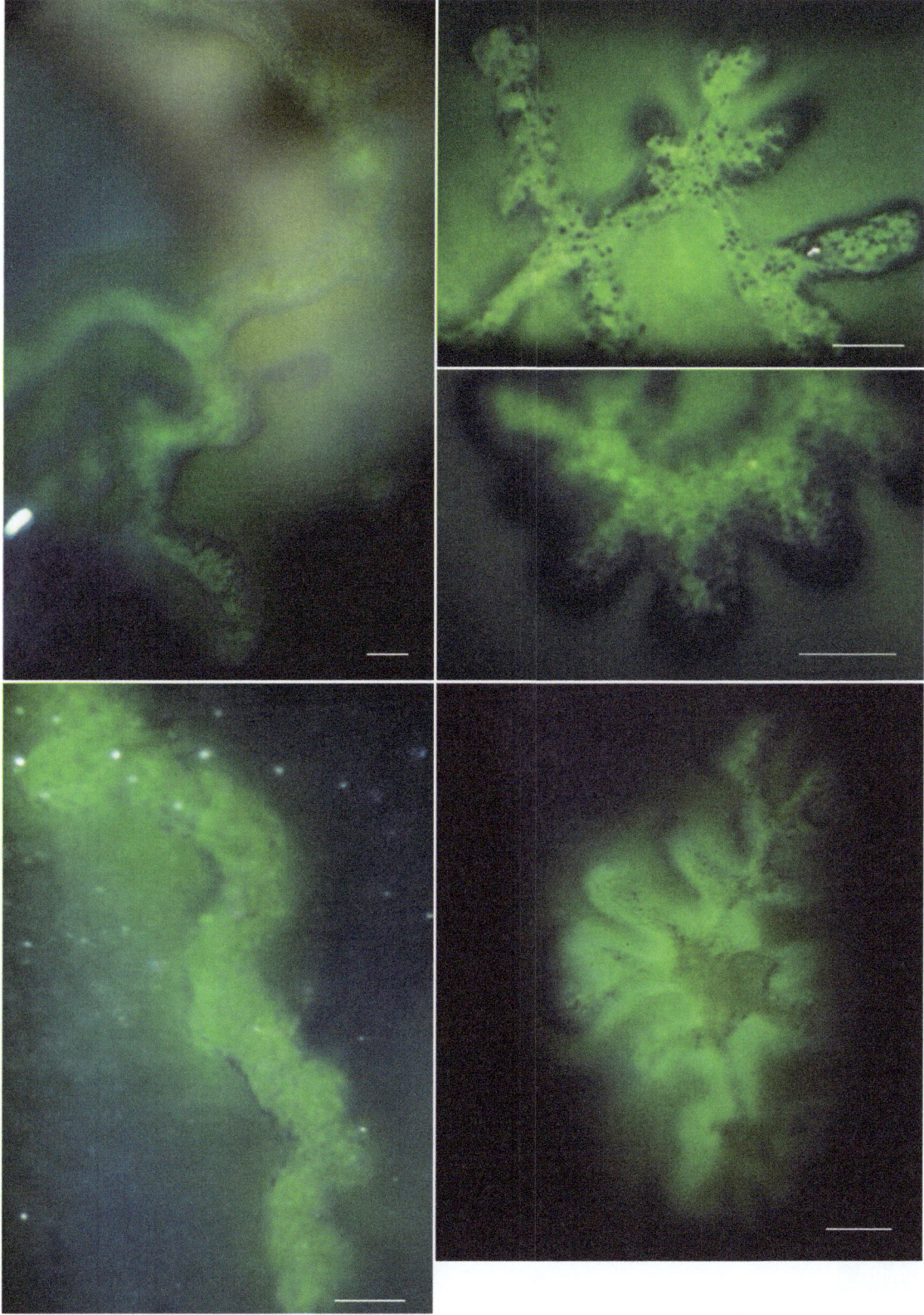

Fig. 1.21 Examples of various shapes of HSV dendritic corneal epithelial figures as visualized with fluorescein sodium

Some Other Shapes of HSV Lesions

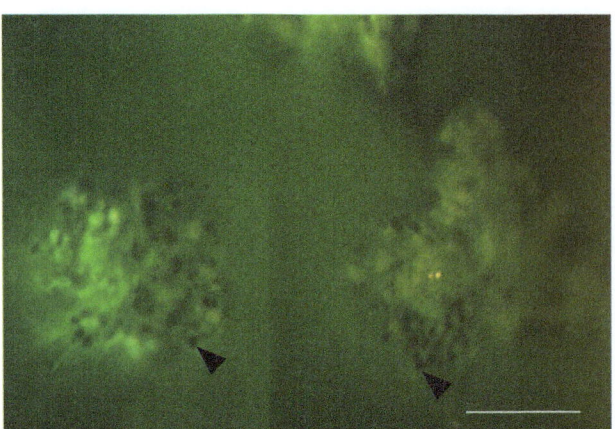

Fig. 1.22 Variously shaped HSV lesions containing swollen/rounded cells (*arrowheads*) (composed photograph)

Comment

This 30-year-old man had a bilateral epithelial keratitis diagnosed as adenovirus infection. The infection left subepithelial opacities. Two months later, he presented with a new epithelial keratitis in the right eye. The correct diagnosis was HSV infection.

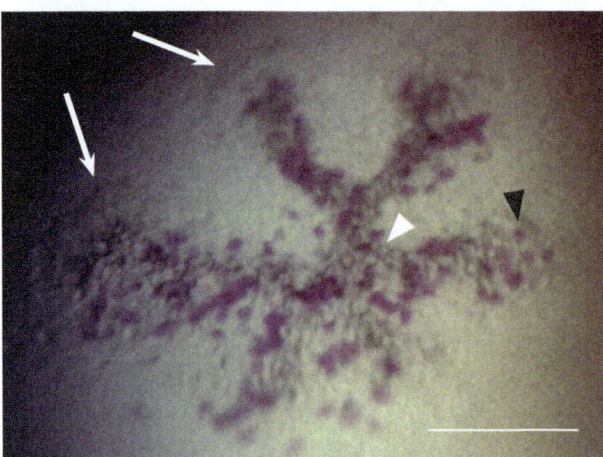

Fig. 1.23 A typical minidendrite showing "terminal bulbs" (rounded enlargements of the branch endings, *arrows*). Some swollen/rounded cells stained red with rose bengal (*black arrowhead*); others did not (*white arrowhead*)

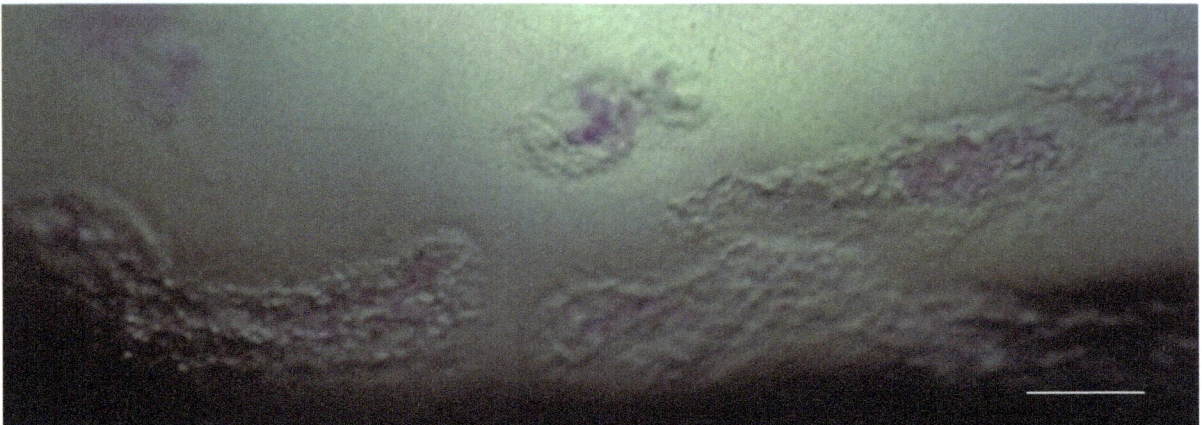

Fig. 1.24 An example of several elongated HSV lesions close to each other. In places, devitalized elements within the lesions stained red with rose bengal

Comment

This 32-year-old woman had no known previous herpetic eye disease. Two days before this photograph was taken, the lesions resembling scratches were misinterpreted as a result of a mechanical injury.

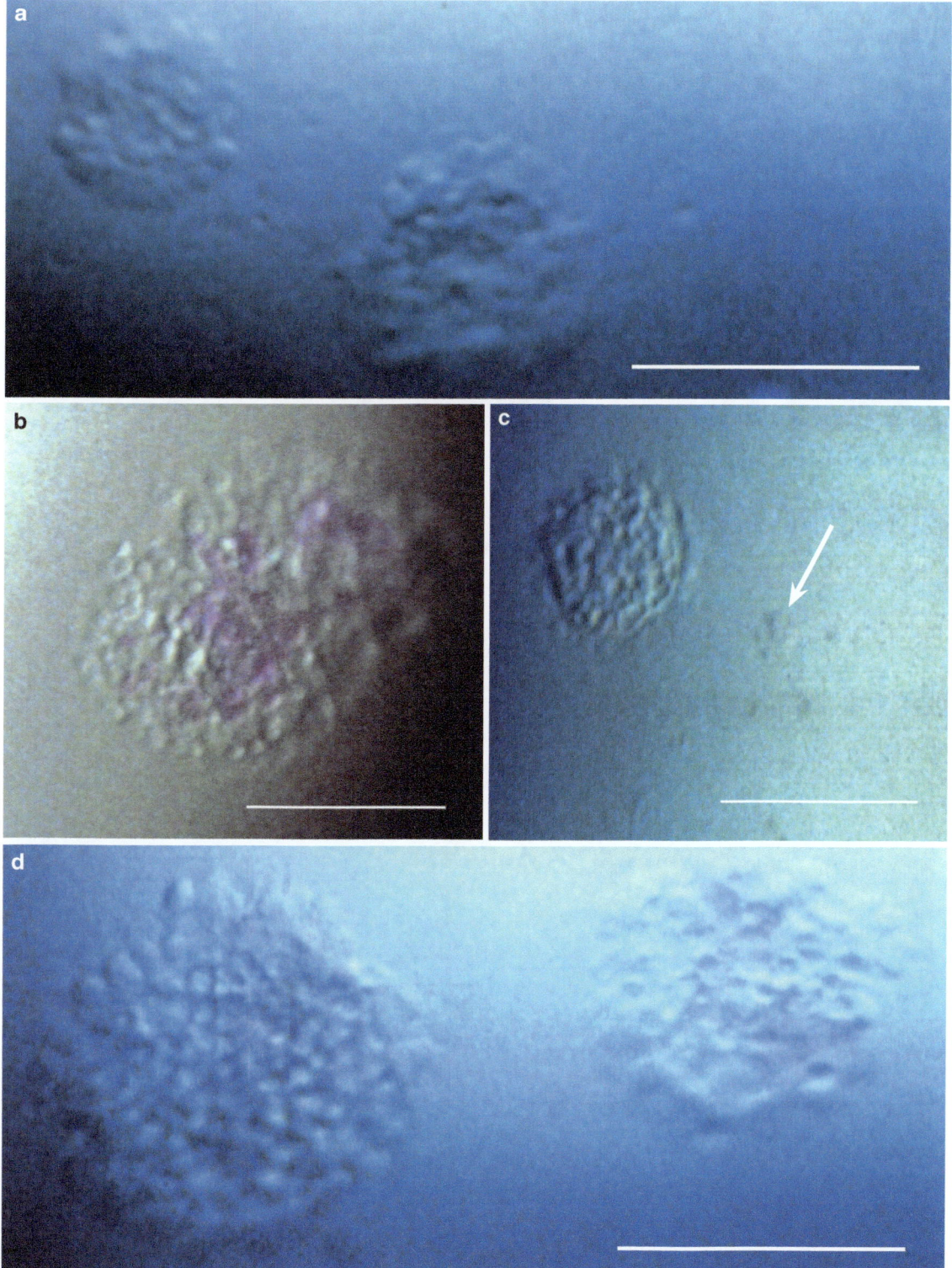

Fig. 1.25 a–d Medallion-like lesions consisting of closely packed swollen/rounded cells. Such lesions are often combined with other HSV lesions, but sometimes a singular one can be the only indication of an HSV infection. (**b**) additionally shows rose bengal staining of a medallion-like lesion and (**c**) incipient cell swelling (*arrow*) close to another such lesion

Precursors of HSV Geographic Lesions

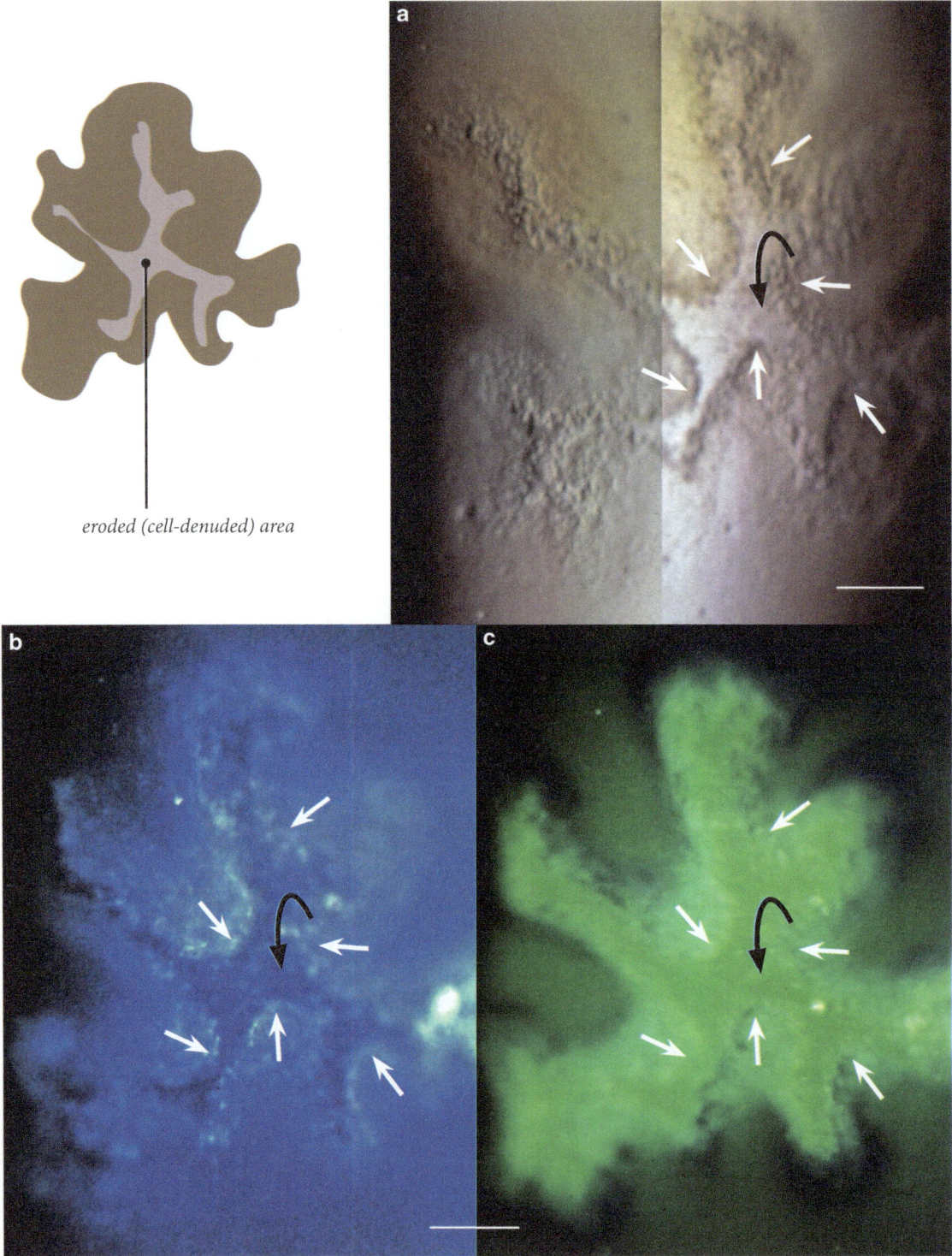

eroded (cell-denuded) area

Fig. 1.26 a–c In this HSV lesion, (**a**) an almost cell-denuded area (*black arrow*) is surrounded by epithelial flaps (*white arrows*; composed photograph). (**b**) The eroded area appears dark; the diseased epithelium is grayish. (**c**) Green-stained tear fluid is pooling within the eroded area and diffusing into and/or below the flaps. The dye is still present in the tear film. A further loss of substance might result in a lesion similar to that shown in Fig. 1.27 (the markers indicate corresponding locations)

HSV Geographic Lesions

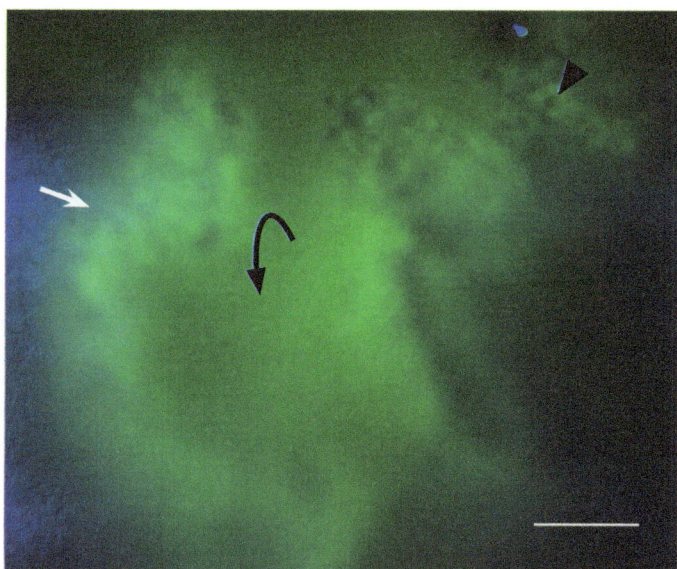

HSV lesions in which a substantial epithelial destruction and loss of substance has occurred often lose their typical configurations. Such lesions are often termed geographic

Fig. 1.27 In this HSV lesion, loss of substance has resulted in epithelial erosion (surface depression), here revealed by pooling of the green-stained tear fluid (*bowed arrow*). The bright green areas (*white arrow*) indicate fluorescein diffusion into the surroundings. Swollen cells at the periphery (*arrowhead*) imply an HSV infection

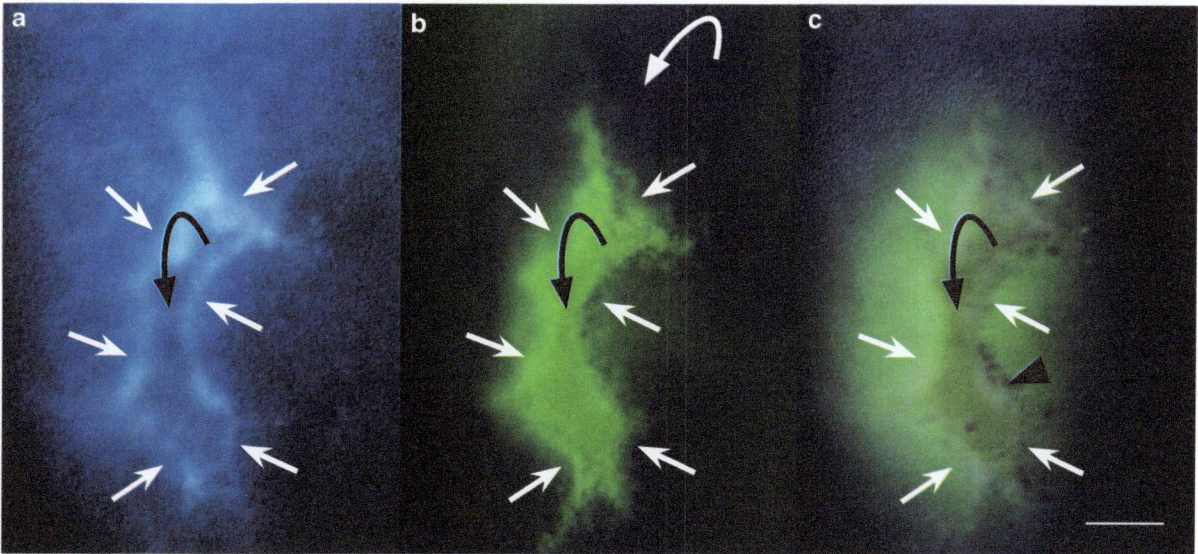

Fig. 1.28 a–c Another example of epithelial erosion caused by HSV (the markers indicate corresponding locations). (**a**) An eroded area (*black bowed arrow*) is surrounded by bright, light-reflecting edges (*white arrows*). (**b**) Tear fluid stained green with fluorescein sodium is pooling within the eroded (depressed) area and diffusing into/below the edges; the presence of fluorescein sodium in the tear film reveals surface elevations in the surroundings (dark areas, *white bowed arrow*). (**c**) After a couple of minutes, more extensive fluorescein diffusion is visible; a few diseased cells stain with rose bengal (*arrowhead*)

Comment

This type of HSV lesion might be difficult to differentiate from healing erosions caused by other injuries, for example mechanical ones.

A Case of Primary HSV Keratitis

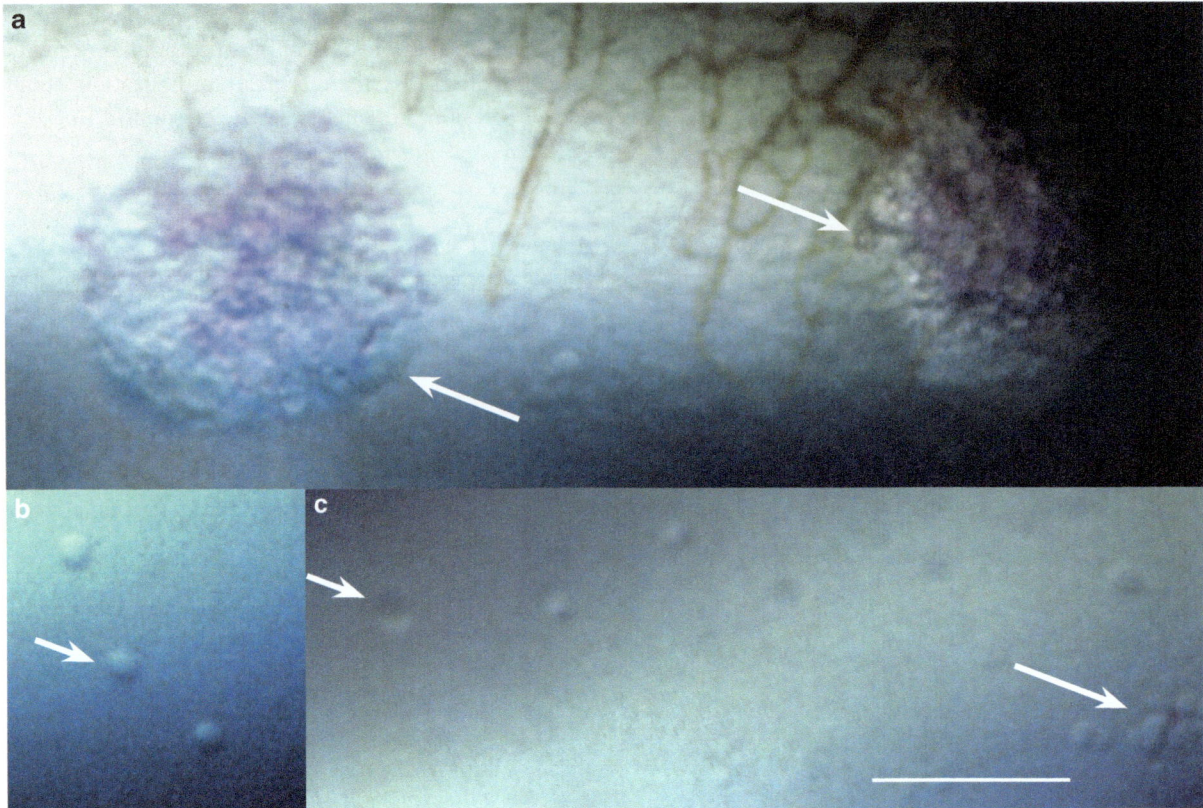

Fig. 1.29 a–c In this case of *primary HSV keratitis*, the corneal epithelium shows (**a**) two rounded lesions at the corneoscleral limbus (*arrows*) and (**b** and **c**) many small clear vesicles (*short arrows*), individual or grouped (**c**, *long arrow*). (Adapted from [6])

Case Report

A 23-year-old soft contact lens wearer presented with a ≤3-day history of increasing irritation in his left eye. Eight days earlier, he had suffered an injury ("collision with someone's head") against the left side of the face and the left eye, and he had lost the left lens. The lens was replaced by his optician 3 days later. The irritation started after 2 days of wearing the lens uneventfully. He stopped using the left lens but continued to use the right one. At presentation, he reported grittiness and purulent discharge from the left eye. The right eye was quiet. The left eye was injected, and the corneal epithelium showed myriad pinpoint lesions spread all over the surface, some staining bright green with fluorescein sodium. Two small rounded foci were present at the upper temporal limbus; one of them seemed partly ulcerated. There was also a small crusted lesion on the lower lid

margin, reported by the patient as present since the accident. The preliminary diagnosis was adenovirus infection. One day later, the lids on the left side were swollen, the preauricular lymph node was tender, and the cornea showed several rounded lesions. After a further 24 h, the patient reported fever, and the epithelial lesions showed propensity to confluence. HSV infection was suspected, and acyclovir treatment (both oral and topical) was started. On the next day, the lid edema had subsided, but the cornea showed branching figures. At this time, the patient reported a slight irritation in the right eye; the eye was slightly injected, and the cornea showed one small rounded epithelial lesion. A virus isolation test in cell culture showed HSV-1. Primary HSV infection was verified by serological tests in paired acute and convalescent sera.

Addendum: HSV Conjunctival Lesions

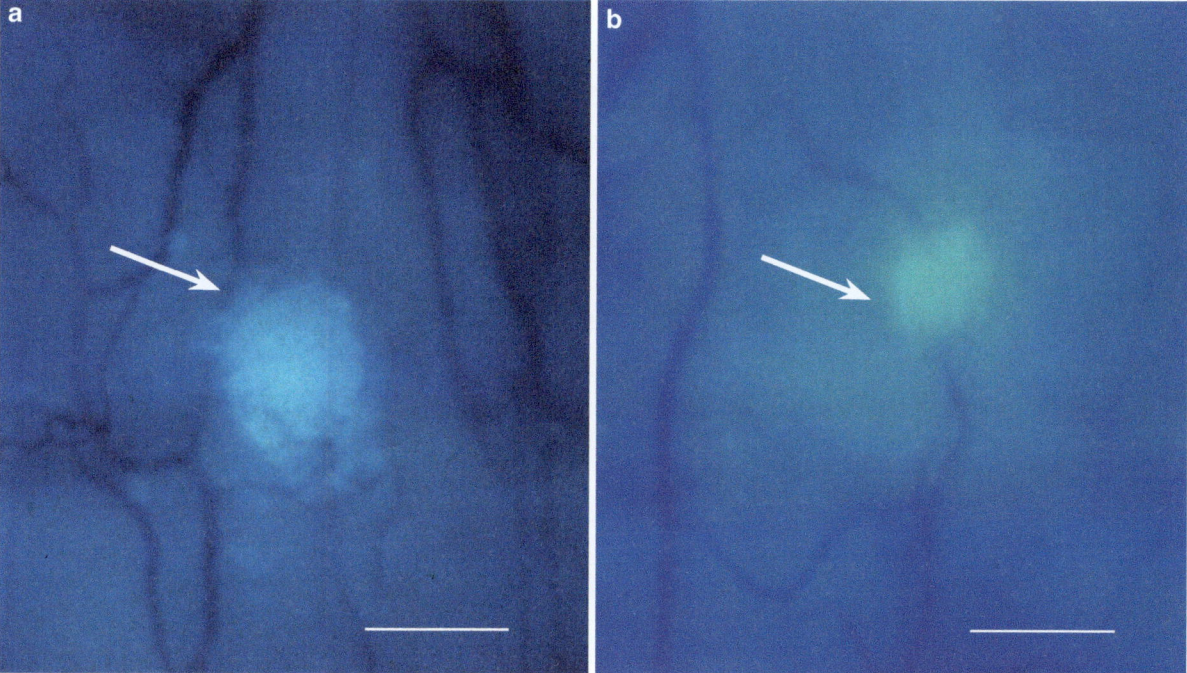

Fig. 1.30 a–b Rounded conjunctival lesions (*arrows*) were the only discernible surface changes in these two patients with HSV infection. Such lesions are difficult to recognize as caused by HSV because they are unspecific (fluorescein sodium, blue filter)

Comment

HSV dendritic conjunctival lesions have been reported. They seem rather rare.

Chapter 2

Healing of Herpes Simplex Virus Epithelial Keratitis Treated with Acyclovir Ointment and Short-Term Sequelae of the Infection

Application of 3% acyclovir ointment five times a day results in a *rapid* (within 24 h) *loss of typical morphological features relatable to HSV infection.* After a further 24 h, some swollen/rounded cells are still visible, but whether they still represent the virus cytopathic effect (CPE) or are an unspecific phenomenon remains open.

Later, the discernible pathology reflects *sequelae* of the infection: scattered *superficial damaged cells* or *confluent cell debris* (staining red with rose bengal), small *cystic spaces* (punctate green fluorescein staining), epithelial *surface elevations* (dark areas in the tear film stained green with fluorescein sodium), and large numbers of *abnormal cells*, located about the level of the basement membrane. At present, lacking histological preparations for comparison, the exact nature of these cells cannot be decided; they might represent damaged cells with altered optical properties or invading inflammatory ones. Of these sequelae, rose bengal and fluorescein sodium staining are first to disappear. The persistence for many months of the abnormal cells, individual or clustered (cf. Chap. 3, Case 2), favors an assumption of inflammatory cells attracted by the virus antigen.

The only known *side effect of acyclovir ointment* is a punctate epithelial keratitis occurring in about 10% of patients. These changes are distinguishable as superimposed on the pathology relatable to HSV infection, and they disappear after the treatment is stopped.

H. M. Tabery, *Herpes Simplex Virus Epithelial Keratitis*
DOI: 978-3-642-01012-5_2, © Springer-Verlag Berlin Heidelberg 2010

Healing of HSV Epithelial Keratitis with Acyclovir Ointment

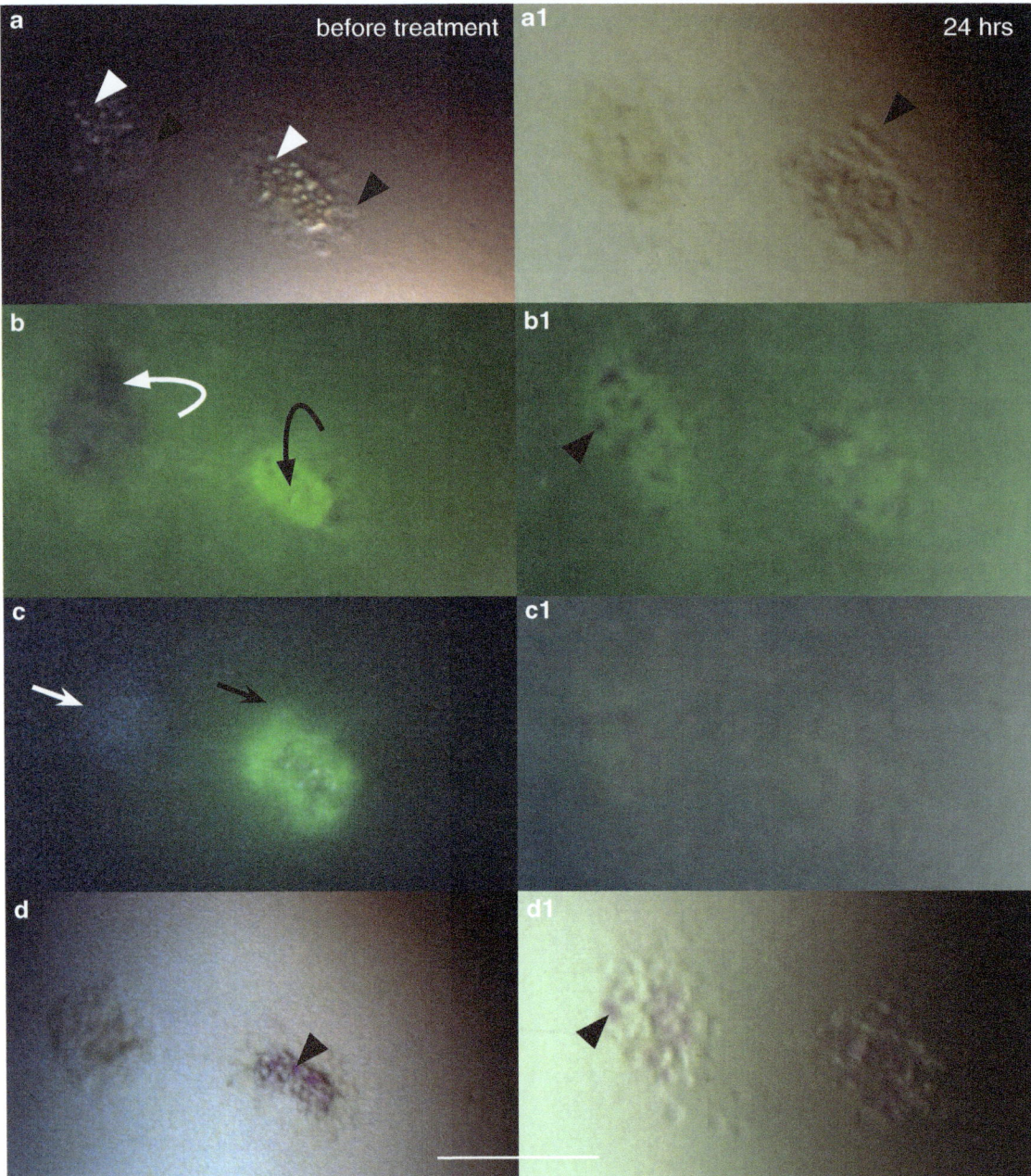

Fig. 2.1 a–d Healing of two small HSV lesions located in the lower part of the cornea (cf. drawing, opposite page)

Left column: At presentation, the lesions showed (**a**) swollen/rounded "bright" cells in the center (*white arrowheads*) and "dull" cells in the surroundings (*black arrowheads*); (**b**) with fluorescein sodium, surface elevation (*white arrow*) or depression (*black arrow*) and (**c**) no diffusion (*white arrow*) or diffusion (*black arrow*); and (**d**) with rose bengal, no staining or a few red dots (*arrowhead*) *Right column:* After *24 h of treatment,* (**a**) some swollen cells (*arrowhead*) are still visible (cf. also **d**), (**b**) some swollen cells are protruding (*arrowhead*) in the green-stained tear fluid, (**c**) there is no diffusion into the tissues, and (**d**) both lesions show weak staining with rose bengal (*arrowhead*)

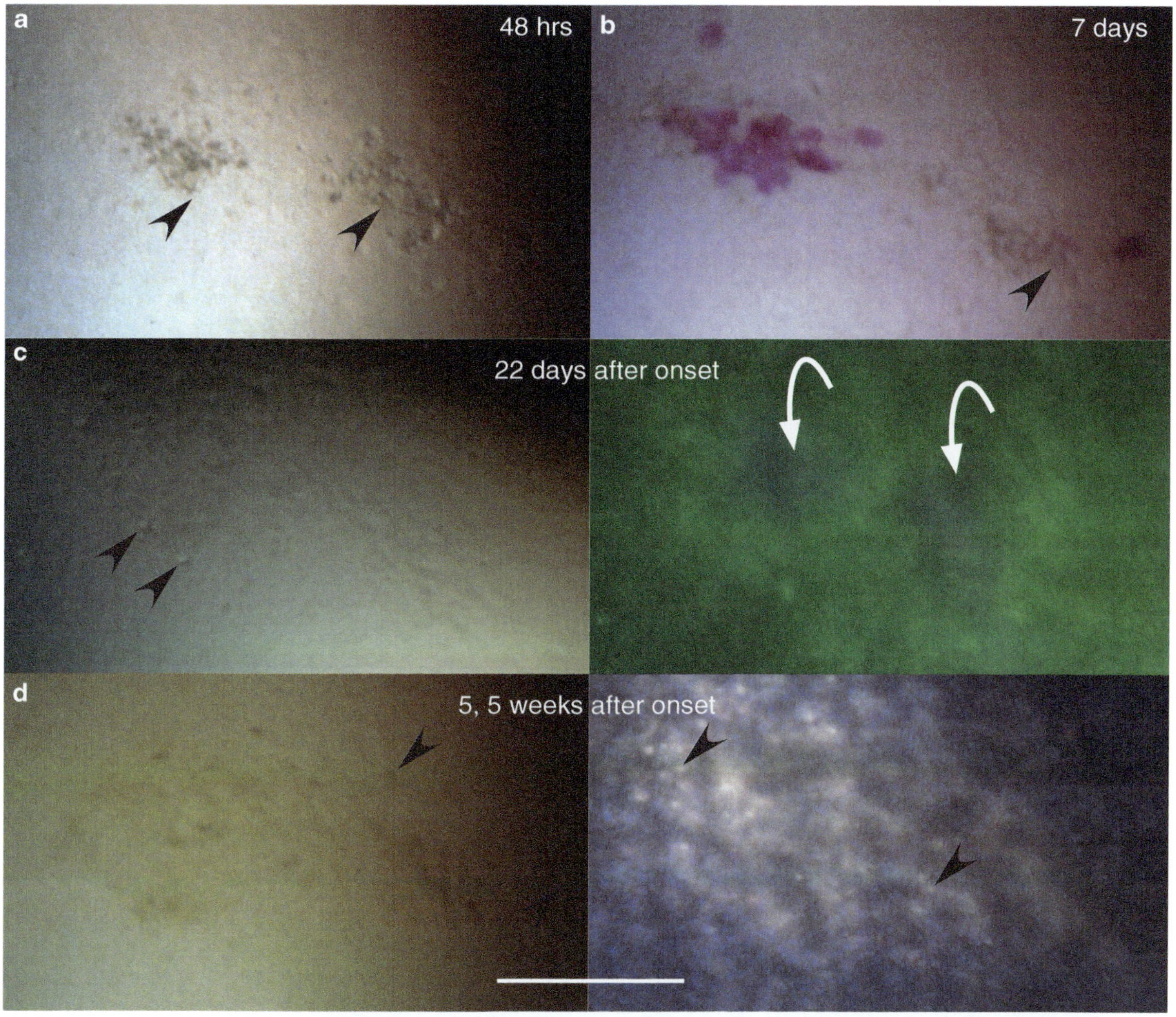

Fig. 2.2 a–d The same two lesions as in Fig. 2.1. Starting after 48 h of treatment, (**a**) the lesions show abnormal cells (a, b, c, d, *arrowheads*) and additional features such as (**b**) patchy red staining with rose bengal after 7 days of treatment. (**c**) Surface elevations (*arrows*) 22 days after onset. (**d**) A subepithelial opacity containing light-reflecting abnormal cells (*arrowheads*) 5.5 weeks after onset

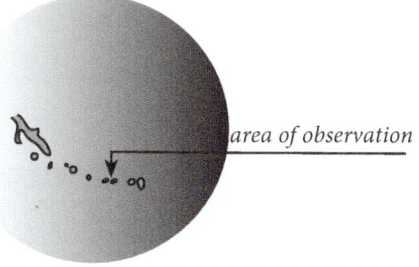

area of observation

Case Report

A 47-year-old woman with recurrent HSV epithelial keratitis in the left eye presented within 24 h of symptoms. The cornea showed a larger lesion and about 10 small ones, arranged in a bowed line running subcentrally from about 9 o'clock toward 4 o'clock (cf. drawing). The patient was treated with acyclovir ointment for 12 days. Nine months after onset, when last seen, the cornea showed fine subepithelial opacities in the locations of the original lesions.

Healing of HSV Epithelial Keratitis with Acyclovir Ointment

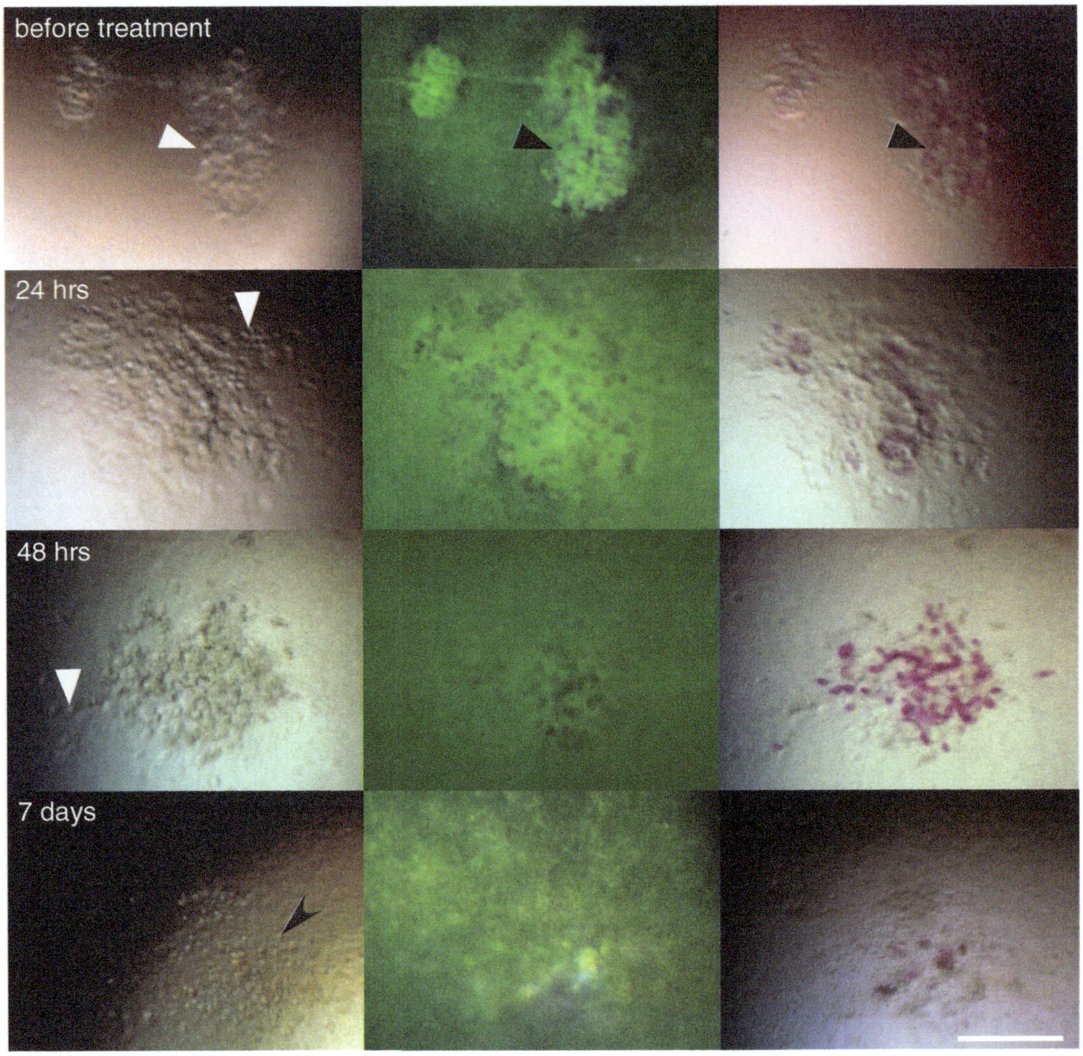

Fig. 2.3 Survey of resolution of two other epithelial lesions in the cornea shown in Figs. 2.1 and 2.2

Left column, without staining: Two adjacent foci containing swollen/rounded cells (*white arrowhead*) floated together within 24 h of treatment and diminished in size within 48 h. Abnormal cells (*black arrowhead*) are visible after 7 days
Middle column, with fluorescein sodium: Green-stained tear fluid is pooling within the lesions; some cells are protruding (dark dots, *arrowhead*). Protruding cells are visible after 24 and 48 h but not after 7 days
Right column, with rose bengal: Some diseased surface cells/cell debris stain red (*arrowhead*). The staining is pronounced after 48 h; only a little staining is present after 7 days

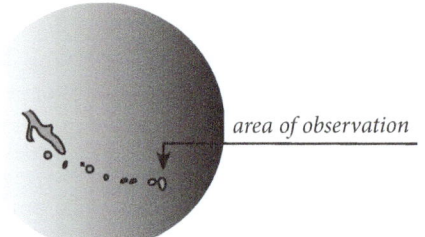

area of observation

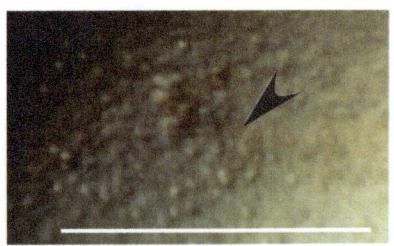

Fig. 2.4 Large numbers of abnormal cells (*arrowhead*) captured after 7 days of treatment

Healing of HSV Epithelial Keratitis with Acyclovir Ointment

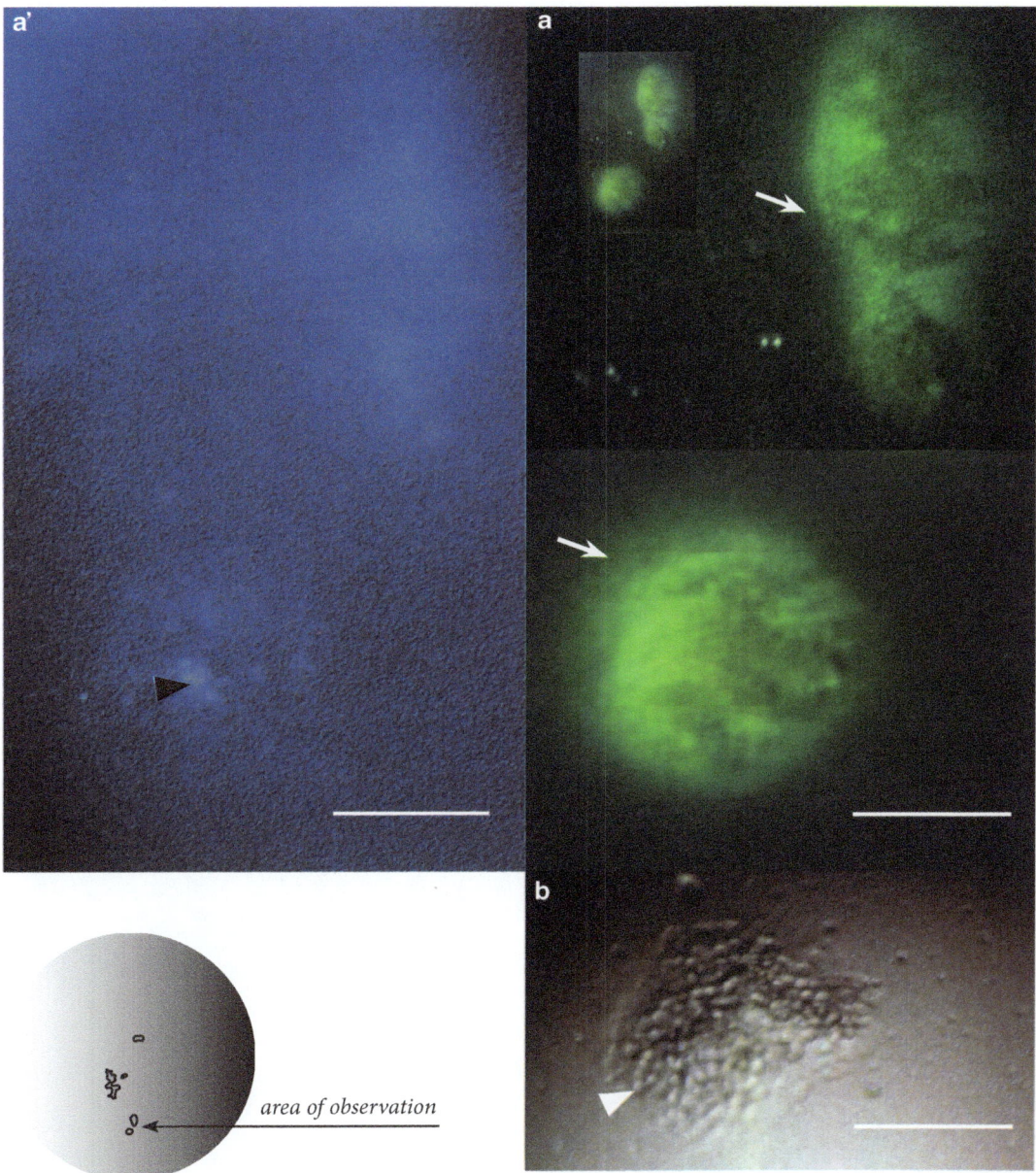

Fig. 2.5 a'–b Two small HSV lesions before treatment. The lesions are located in the lower part of the cornea (cf. drawing). Their rose bengal staining is shown in Fig. 2.6 and their resolution in Figs. 2.7–2.9. (**a'**) Before staining, the lesions appear as gray shadows. Some light-reflecting damaged cells show as grayish dots (*black arrowhead*). (**a**) The lesions stain green with fluorescein sodium. The bright green hue indicates fluorescein diffusion into the surroundings (*arrows*; composed photograph). *Inset*: The same area captured in one photograph. (**b**) The lesions contain large numbers of swollen/rounded cells (*arrowhead*); this example shows the lower lesion

Case Report

A 24-year-old man with recurrent HSV keratitis in his left eye since childhood. The duration of symptoms was ≤29 h. The cornea showed a small dendritic figure and four smaller lesions. He was treated with acyclovir ointment five times daily for 10 days.

Healing of HSV Epithelial Keratitis with Acyclovir Ointment

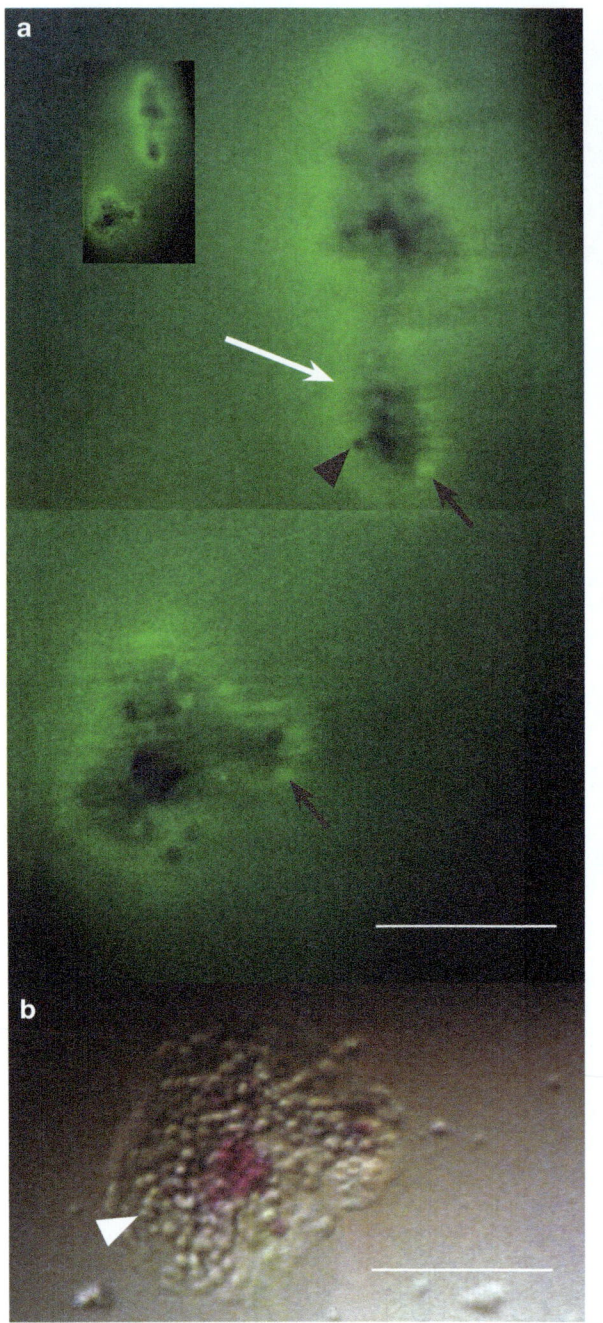

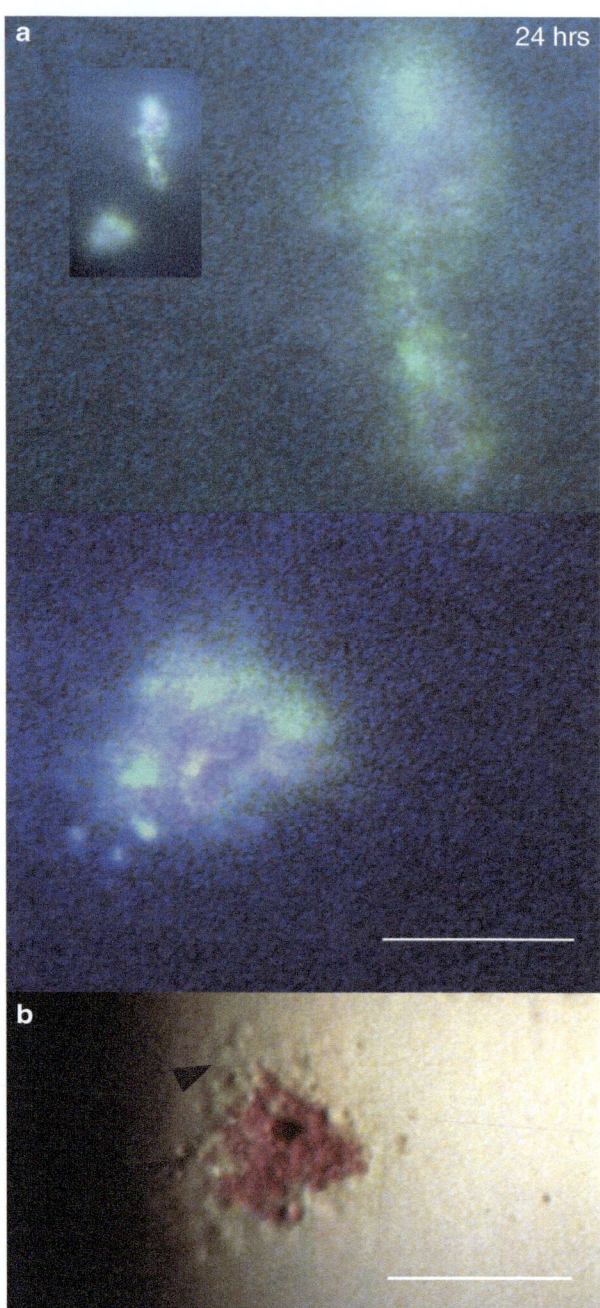

Fig. 2.6 a–b The same lesions as in Fig. 2.5 a few minutes later and after application of rose bengal dye. (**a**) There is extensive fluorescein diffusion into the surroundings (cf. *inset*). The peripheral parts of the lesions show a bright green hue (*white arrow*); bright green dots (*black arrows*) are suggestive of cystic spaces. A few diseased cells stain with rose bengal (*arrowhead*). (**b**) Patchy rose bengal staining present in the lower lesion; the majority of the swollen/rounded cells (*arrowhead*) did not stain. (Adapted from [7])

Fig. 2.7 a–b *After 24 h of treatment* with acyclovir ointment five times a day, the same lesions appear smaller. (**a**) Fluorescein diffusion is limited to the lesions. There is patchy staining with rose bengal. (**b**) Patchy rose bengal staining visualizes surface debris. Structures indicated by *arrowheads* represent either swollen/rounded cells or small cysts. (Adapted from [7])

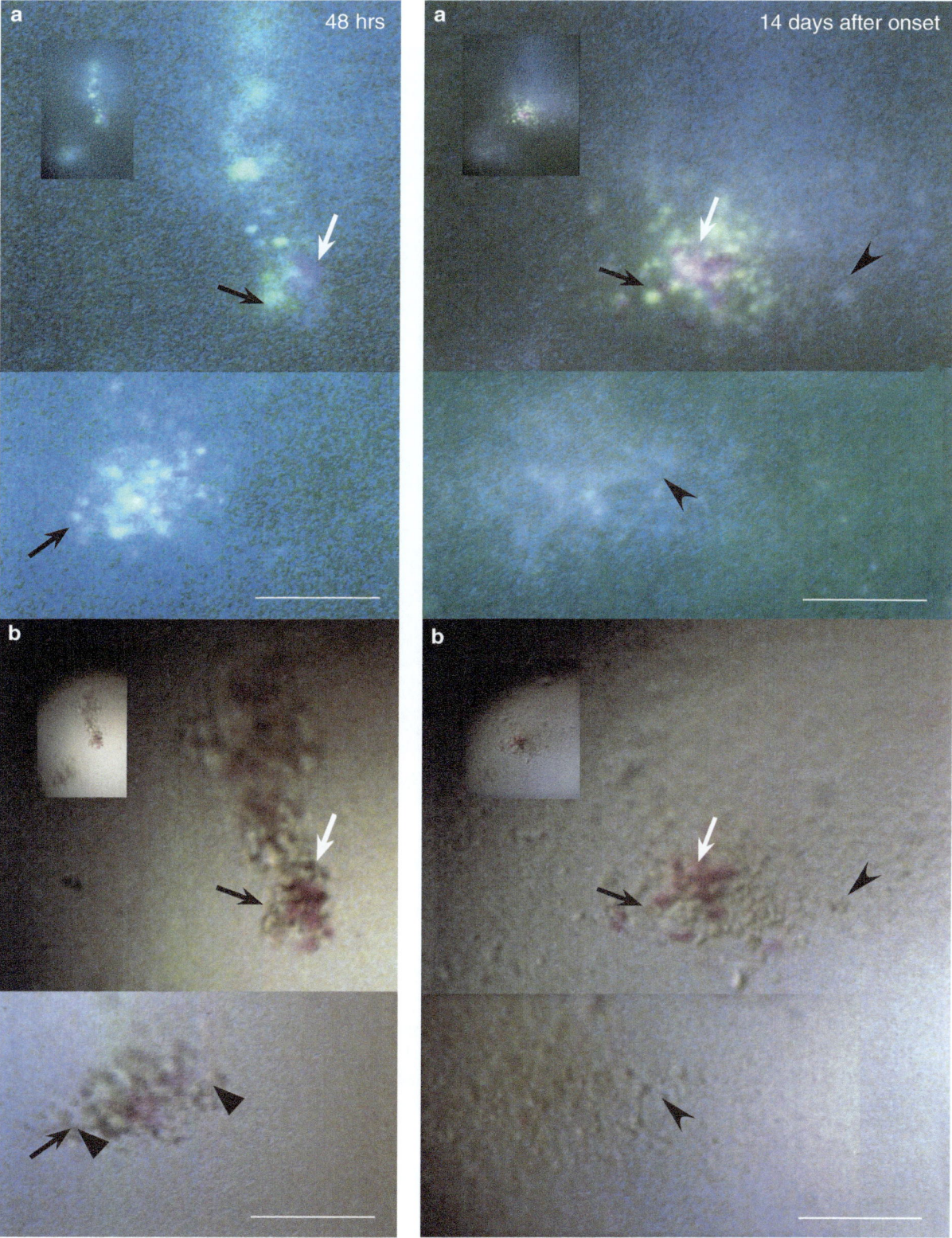

Fig. 2.8 a–b Seen after *48 h of treatment* are small cystic spaces (*black arrows*), patchy rose bengal staining (*white arrows*), and swollen/rounded cells or small cysts (*arrowheads*). (Adapted from [7])

Fig. 2.9 a–b *Two weeks after onset.* Small cystic spaces (*black arrows*), patchy rose bengal staining (*white arrows*), and accumulated light-reflecting abnormal cells (*arrowheads*). For close view, see Fig. 2.11, overleaf (the markers are placed in corresponding locations)

Healing of HSV Epithelial Keratitis with Acyclovir Ointment

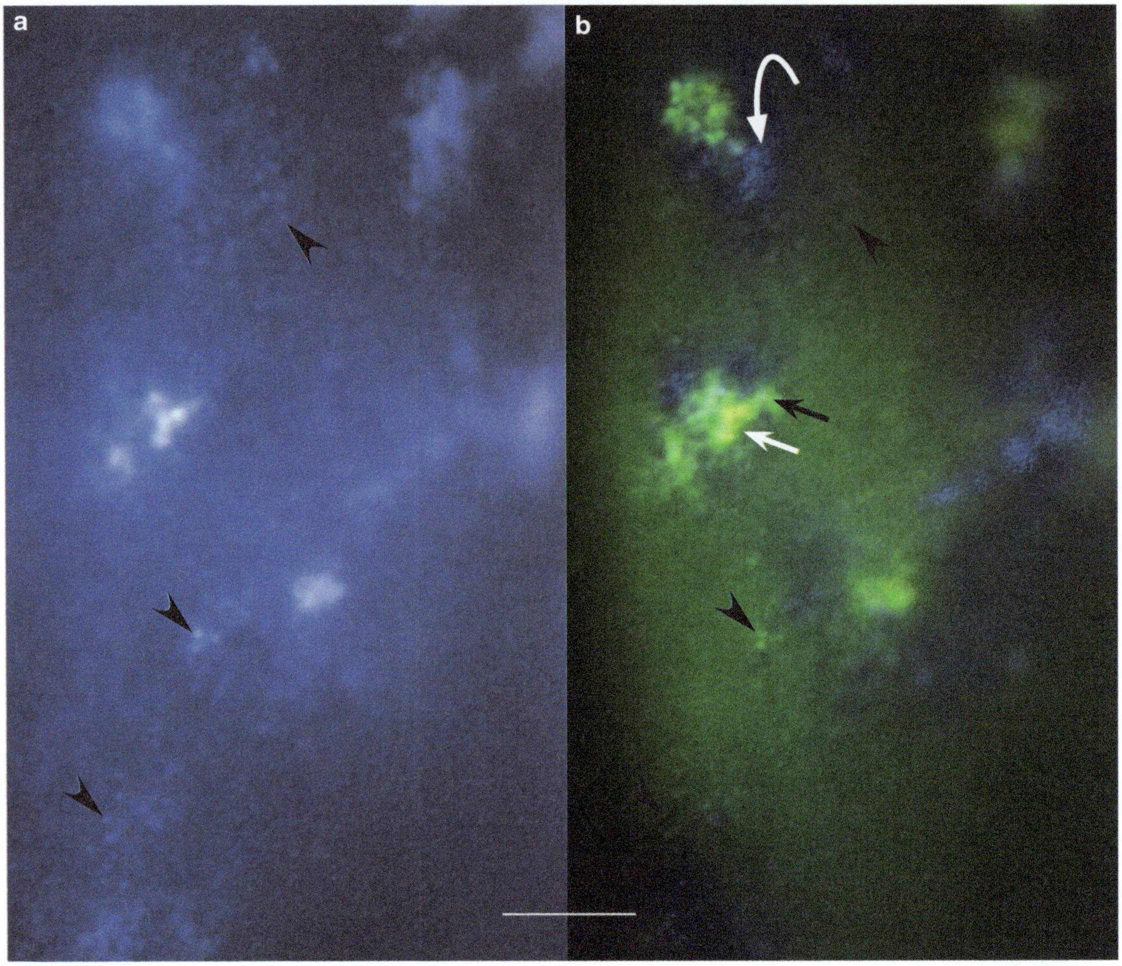

Fig. 2.10 a–b After 7 days of treatment with acyclovir ointment, the branching configuration of a classic dendritic lesion is still well discerned. (**a**) Before staining, the involved area shows many light-reflecting abnormal cells (*arrowheads*). (**b**) Fluorescein sodium reveals cystic spaces (*black arrow*) and surface elevations (*bowed arrow*). Abnormal cells (*arrowheads*) are more difficult to discern in the green-stained tear film. Diseased surface cells stain yellow (*white arrow*) with (adherent) fluorescein. (*Arrowheads* in **a** and **b** are placed in corresponding locations)

Case Report

A 66-year-old man with sixth recurrence of HSV epithelial keratitis within 5 years presented after 6 days of irritation and redness in the left eye. The temporal cornea showed a classic dendritic figure and two small lesions close to the upper limbus (cf. drawing). He was treated with acyclovir ointment five times daily for 10 days.

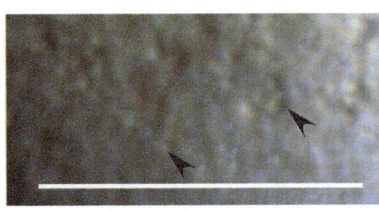

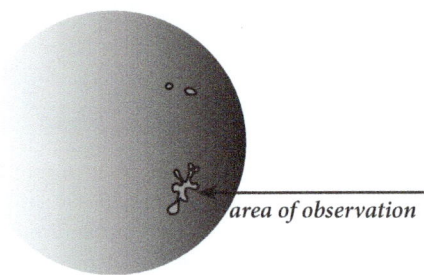

Fig. 2.11 Large numbers of abnormal cells (*arrowheads*) (close view, from Fig. 2.9)

area of observation

Healing of HSV Epithelial Keratitis with Acyclovir Ointment: A Treatment Failure

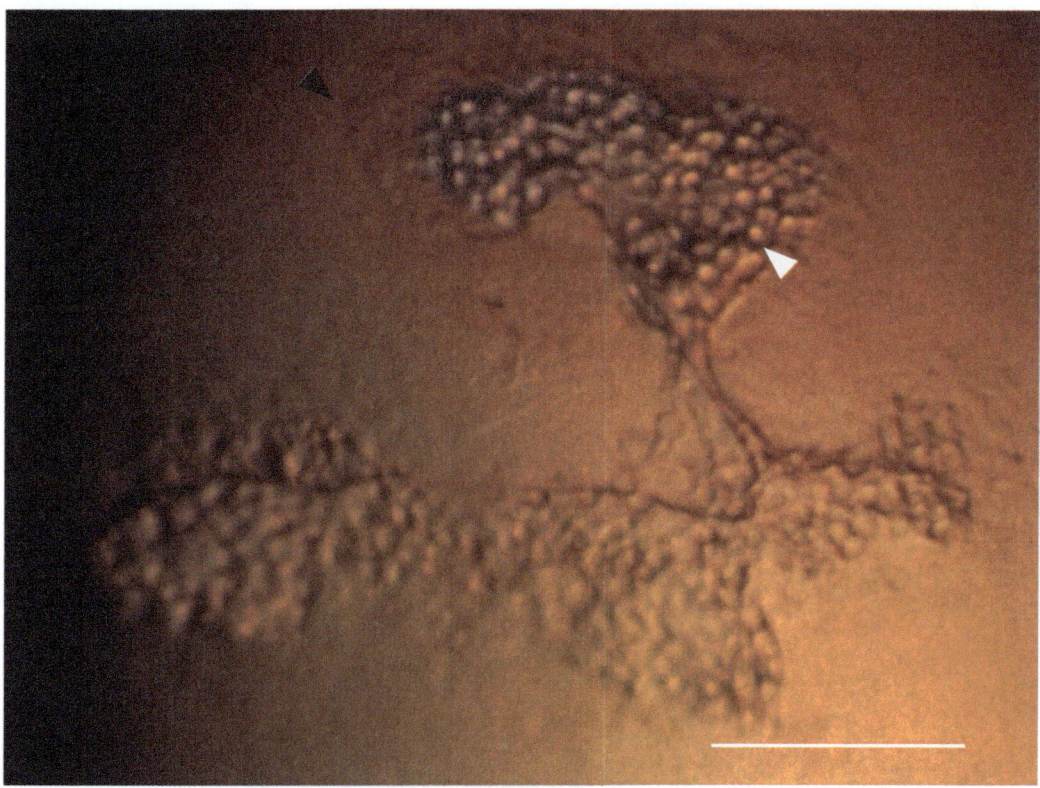

Fig. 2.12 This HSV lesion, (presumably) treated with acyclovir ointment for a week shows typical features of ongoing infection: large numbers of clearly visible "bright" swollen/rounded cells (*white arrowhead*) surrounded by "dull" ones (*black arrowhead*)

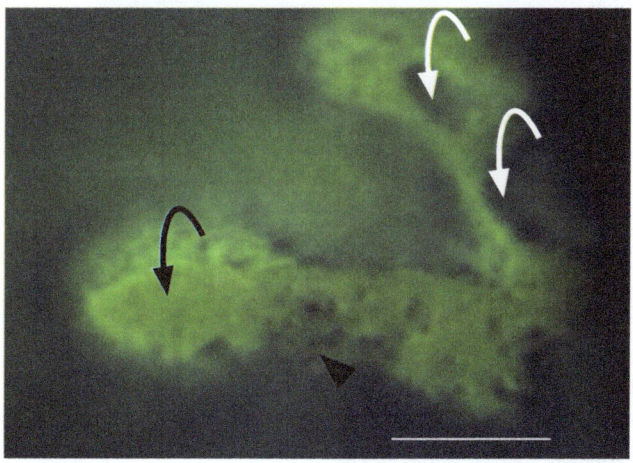

Fig. 2.13 The same lesion as in Fig. 2.12. Tear fluid stained green with fluorescein sodium is pooling in surface depressions (*black arrow*); elevated areas appear dark (*white arrows*). Some swollen cells are visible in the lower part of the lesion (*arrowhead*) (the upper part is slightly out of focus)

Case Report

The patient was a 34-year-old woman with recurrent HSV infections around her left eye. She did not recall any previous eye involvement. Probably, she had not used the ointment properly. She was instructed how to apply it, and a week later all signs of active infection were gone.

Side Effects of Acyclovir Ointment

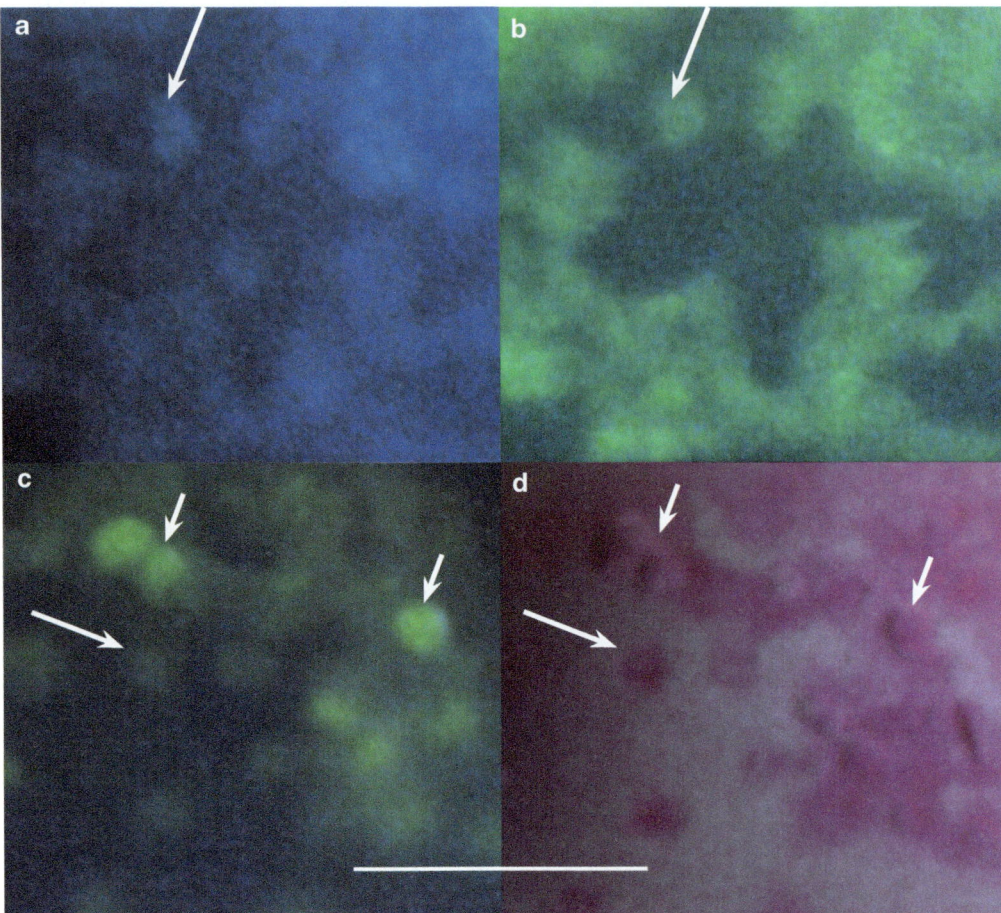

Fig. 2.14 a–d After 7 days of treatment of HSV lesions with acyclovir ointment, the epithelium in the lower part of the cornea shows changes referable to neither the infection nor the healing process. (**a**) Diseased (grayish) surface cells (*arrow*). (**b**) Green staining with fluorescein sodium of the same cells (*arrow*). (**c**) Green staining with fluorescein sodium of diseased cells (*long arrow*) and a brilliant green staining of cystic spaces (*short arrows*). (**d**) Red staining with rose bengal. Both diseased cells (*long arrow*) and the roofs of the cystic spaces (*short arrows*) stain red (cf. **c**). (Adapted from [7])

Comment

All these changes disappeared after the treatment was stopped.

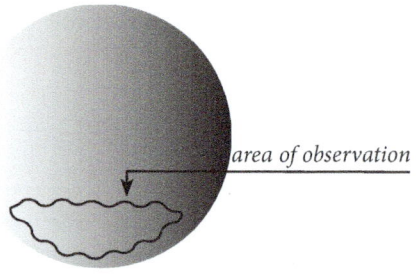

area of observation

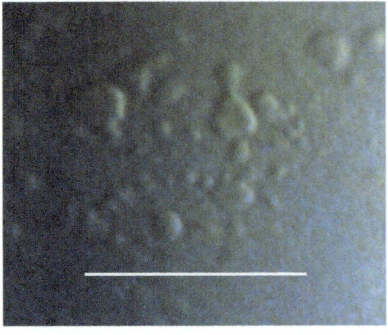

Fig. 2.15 Smaller and larger cystic spaces visible without staining in the same cornea (adjacent to the area shown in Fig. 2.14**c**). (Adapted from [7])

Chapter 3

Complications, Accompanying Signs, Recurrences, and Long-Term Sequelae of Herpes Simplex Virus Epithelial Keratitis

It is rare to see, in the same cornea, two HSV epithelial lesions at different stages of development, that is, one showing signs of *spontaneous healing* and a fresh one (Case 1). Their contemporaneous presence implies two episodes of virus shedding occurring some days apart (about 12 days as judged from the patient's history in this case). This case also shows morphological features of epithelial breakdown sometimes occurring after primary healing of HSV epithelial lesions. Cases 2–5 demonstrate the *pattern of recurring HSV keratitis in different forms.* In the absence of other signs, the herpetic origin of *stromal infiltrates* is difficult to recognize (Case 3). Anterior uveitis with *keratic precipitates* (Case 2) and a *fine epithelial edema* in adjacent areas (Case 4) sometimes accompanies HSV epithelial keratitis. Patients with dry eye may show epithelial lesions exceptionally *heavily stained with rose bengal* (Cases 4 and 5). Long-term sequelae of HSV epithelial keratitis are *subepithelial opacities* ("ghost" figures), some still showing many abnormal cells after 10 months (Case 2). The opacities slowly clear but may remain discernible for many years (17 years after onset, Case 2). Deeper stromal opacities are not a sequela of epithelial keratitis but the result of stromal inflammation (Case 5).

H. M. Tabery, *Herpes Simplex Virus Epithelial Keratitis*
DOI: 978-3-642-01012-5_3, © Springer-Verlag Berlin Heidelberg 2010

Case 1. HSV Epithelial Keratitis: A Fresh and an Older Lesion

Case Report

A 44-year-old man with a history of recurrent herpes labialis but no known herpetic eye disease had irritation in his right eye for 2 weeks. He presented because of worsening of symptoms for 2 days. The cornea showed two branching figures, one located almost centrally and the other one more peripherally (cf. drawing).

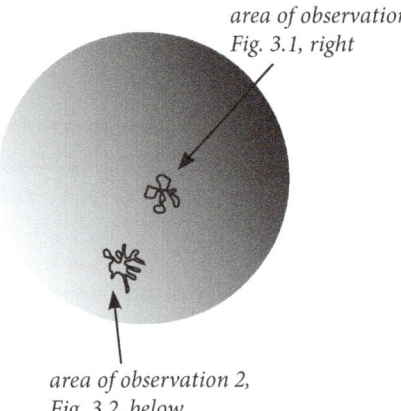

area of observation 1, Fig. 3.1, right

area of observation 2, Fig. 3.2, below

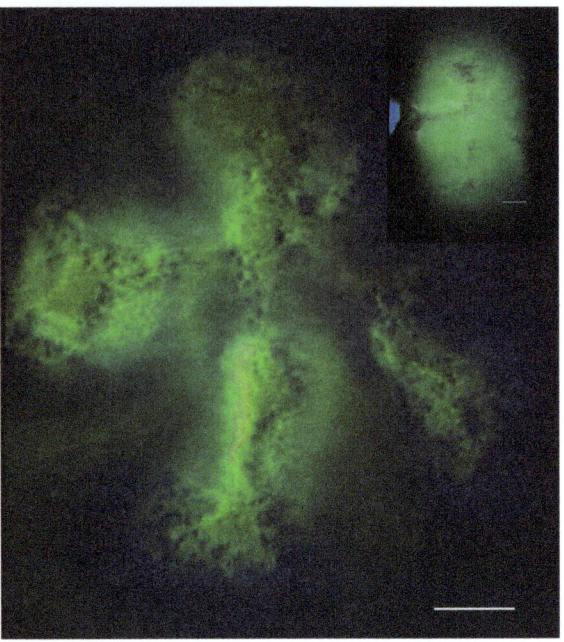

Fig. 3.1 A branching figure with typical features of a fresh HSV infection (cf. Chap. 1). *Inset*: A couple of minutes later, the lesion shows massive fluorescein diffusion

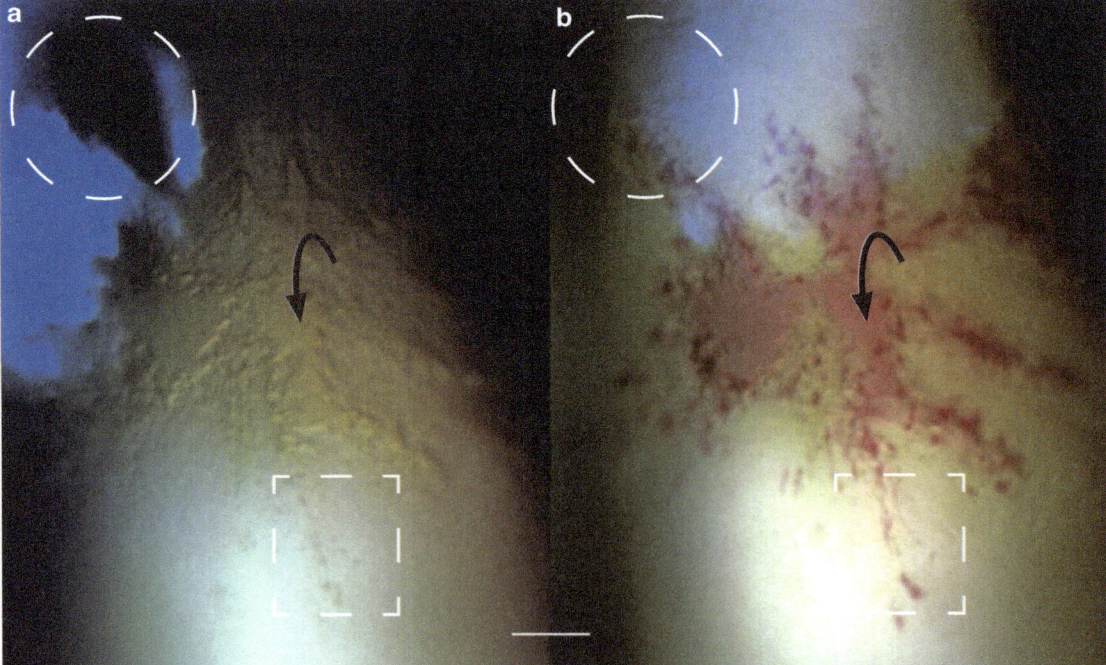

Fig. 3.2 a–b The extensive epithelial destruction resulting in a cell-denuded bottom of the wound (*arrow*) implies an older lesion; the bottom of the erosion and some diseased cells stain red with rose bengal. Spontaneous healing seems to have started at the periphery (in frames). For details, see Fig. 3.3 (circular frame cf. Fig. 3.3a, rectangular frame cf. Fig. 3.3b). (Adapted from [7])

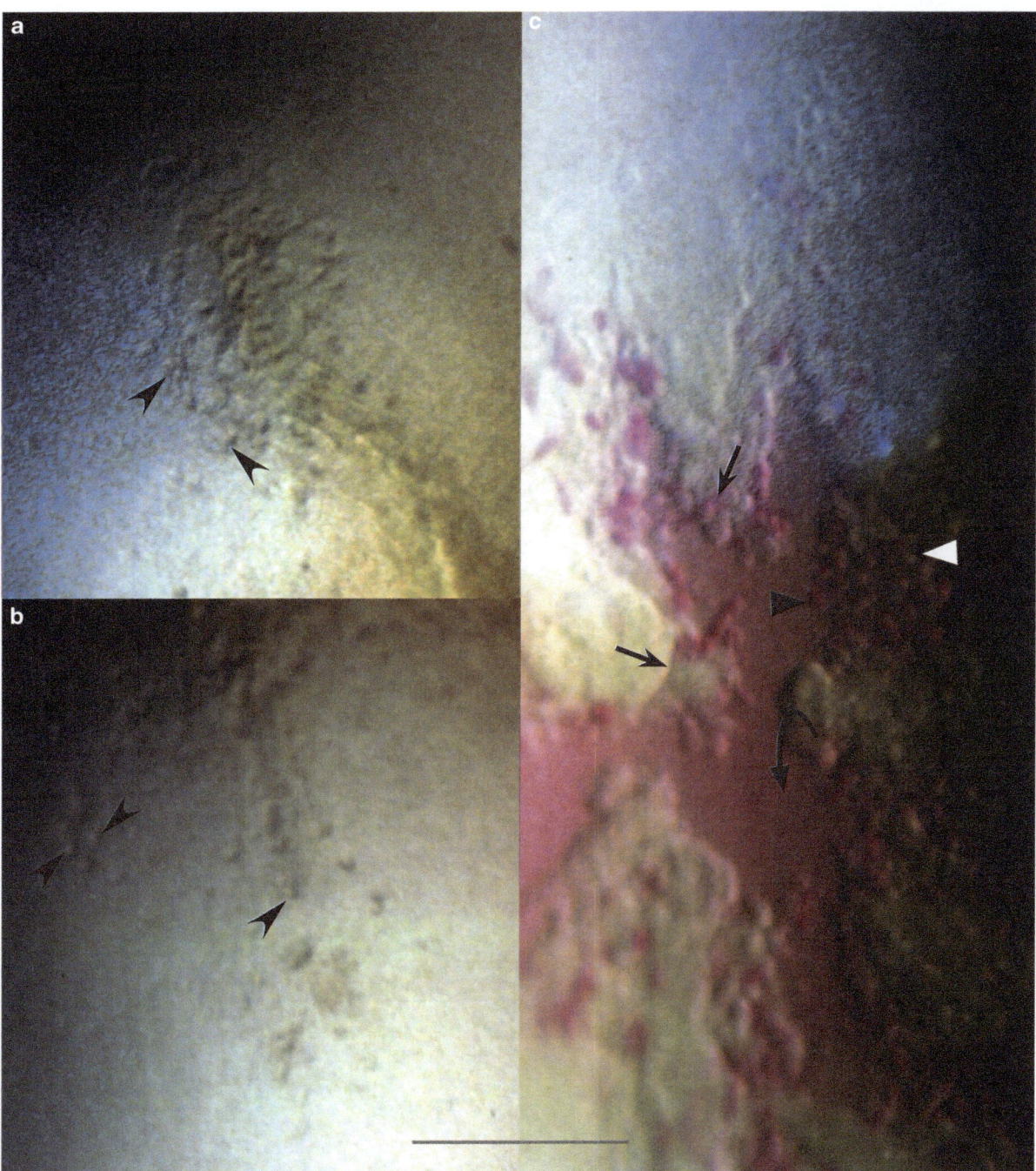

Fig. 3.3 a–c Close view of the lesion shown in Fig. 3.2. (**a**) Spontaneous healing seems to have occurred in the periphery of the left upper branch of the lesion (indicated by the circular frame in Fig. 3.2); similarly to acyclovir-treated lesions (Chap. 2), this area shows many abnormal cells (*arrowheads*). (**b**) A similar phenomenon is visible in the lower branch of the lesion (indicated by the rectangular frame in Fig. 3.2); *arrowheads* indicate abnormal cells. (**c**) The central part of the lesion has a cell-denuded bottom staining red with rose bengal (*bowed arrow*); it is surrounded by rugged edges of epithelial flaps (*short arrows*). The epithelium surrounding the wound bottom shows swollen cells staining (*black arrowhead*) or not staining (*white arrowhead*) with rose bengal. (Adapted from [7])

Comment

The exact nature of the cells shown in (c) (virus-infected ones, representing an unspecific reaction, or both) remains open.

Healing Followed by Epithelial Breakdown and a New Repair (Case 1, cont.)

The patient was treated with acyclovir ointment five times a day. A week later, the cornea showed ghost figures.

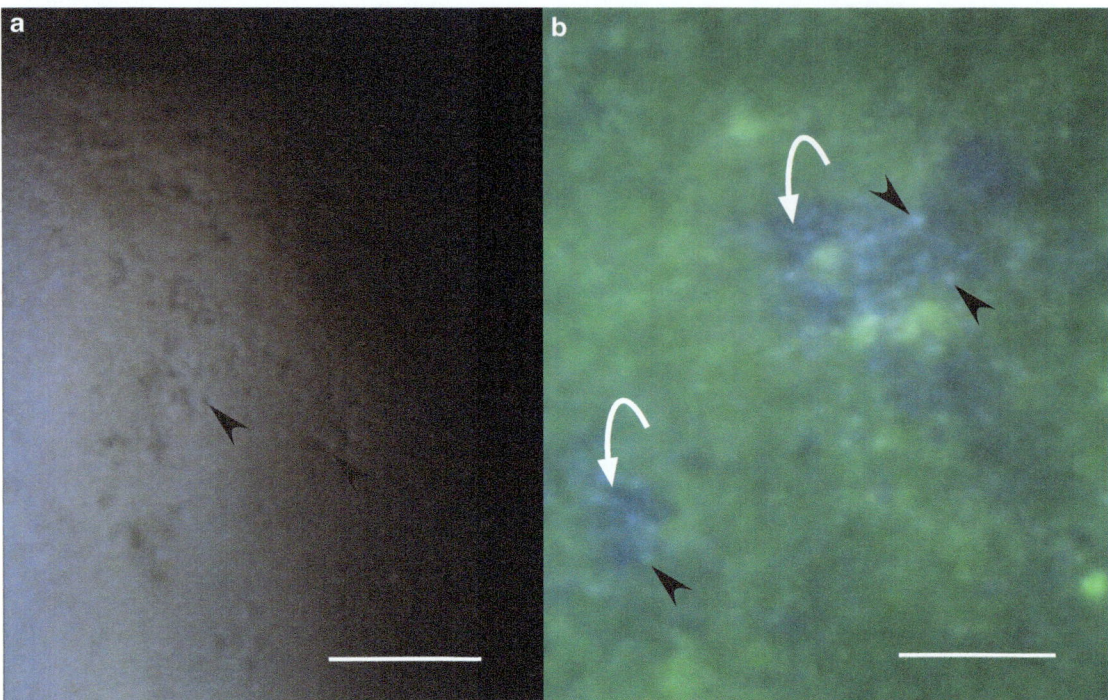

Fig. 3.4 a–b Abnormal cells visible in (**a**) and (**b**) (*arrowheads*) and surface elevations (*arrows*) in (**b**) are regular features of newly healed HSV lesions (Chap. 2). The sites of the (**a**) older and (**b**) the fresh lesion are shown after a week's treatment with acyclovir ointment

After an additional week, the patient presented again because of a new irritation in the same eye. The site of the older lesion showed epithelial breakdown resulting in epithelial ulceration.

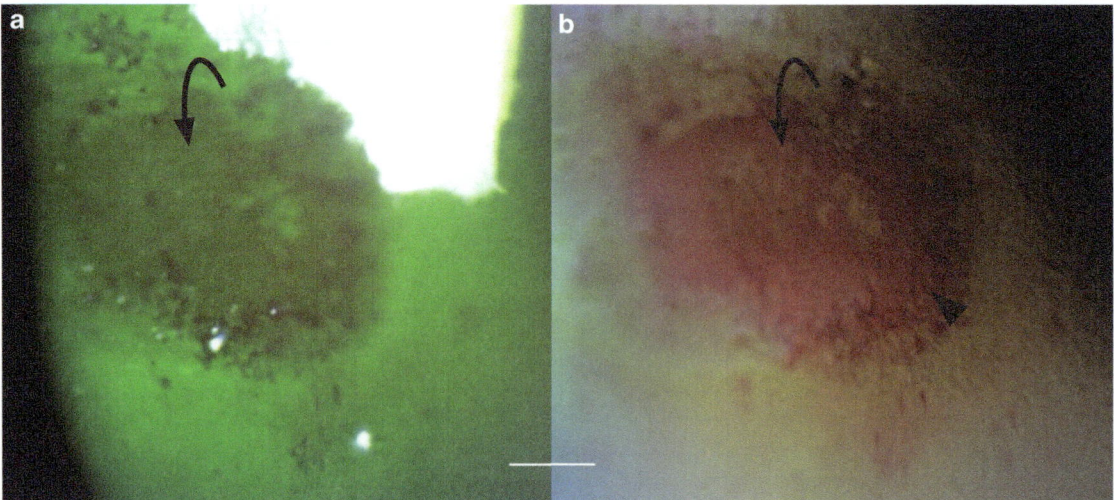

Fig. 3.5 a–b The bottom (*arrows*) of the epithelial ulceration stains red with rose bengal; it seems largely cell-denuded. The edges contain swollen cells (*arrowhead*), the nature of which is difficult to decide. (**a**) A massive fluorescein diffusion into the surroundings is seen (the *arrows* are placed in corresponding locations)

Possibly, the ulceration was sterile; nevertheless, in this particular patient, it was treated with acyclovir ointment five times a day. The healing was slow.

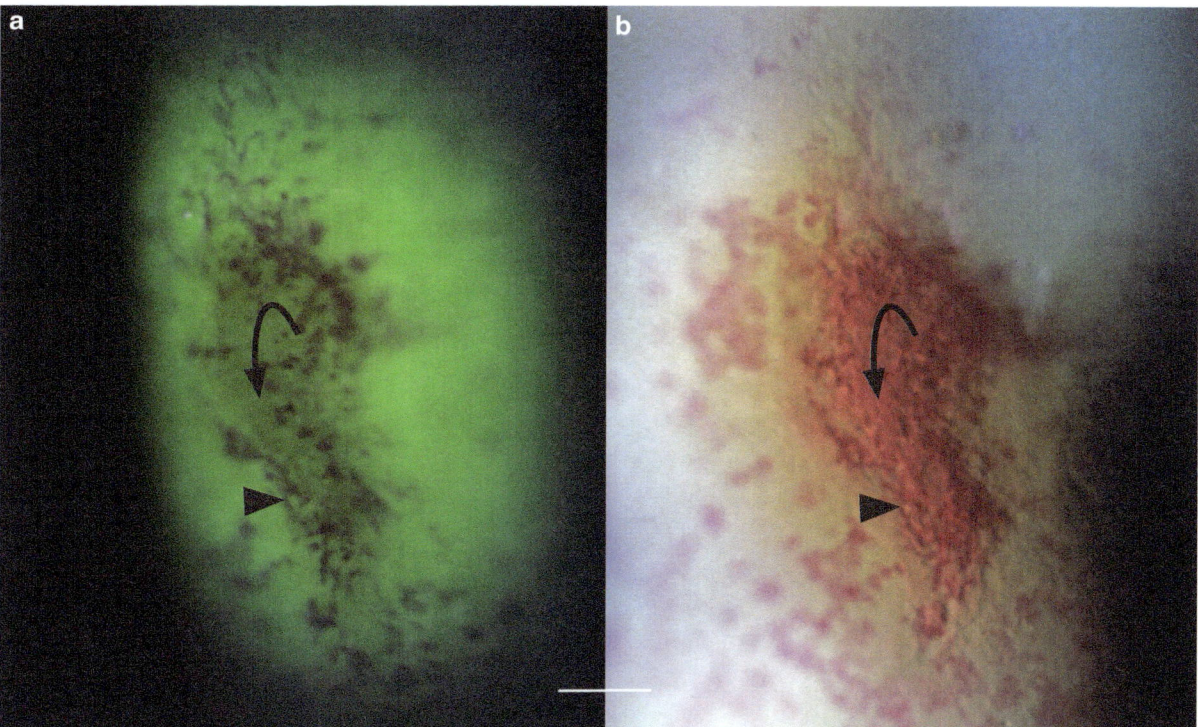

Fig. 3.6 a–b After 5 days of treatment, the epithelial ulceration is smaller (cf. Fig. 3.5). (**a**) There is still massive fluorescein diffusion into the surroundings. (**b**) Swollen epithelial cells (*arrowhead*) now probably represent an unspecific phenomenon. The bottom of the wound (*arrow*) stains red with rose bengal. The surroundings show rose bengal-stained superficial cells (probably a side effect of acyclovir, Chap. 2) (the markers are placed in corresponding locations)

The lesion healed within a further week.

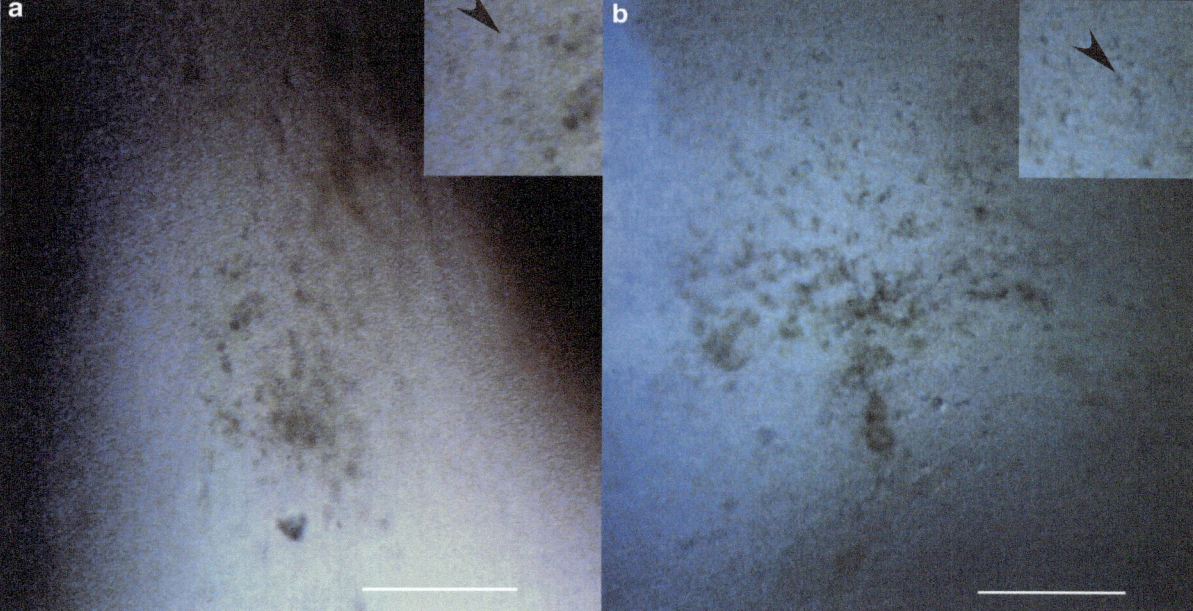

Fig. 3.7 a–b The sites of (**a**) the older lesion and (**b**) the fresh one both show abnormal cells (*insets, arrowhead*) 29 (**a**) and 42 (**b**) days after the first visit

Case 2. Healing of HSV Epithelial Keratitis, Accompanying Signs, and Sequelae

Case Report

A 72-year-old woman with severe visual impairment in her right eye (caused by macular degeneration) presented with HSV epithelial keratitis in her left eye. The duration of symptoms was 7 days. She was treated with acyclovir ointment five times a day for 2 weeks. The photographic observation period was 10 months. She was followed clinically for a further 16 years.

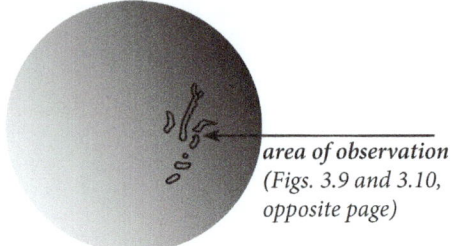

area of observation (Figs. 3.9 and 3.10, opposite page)

Location on the cornea of the lesions shown in Fig. 3.8

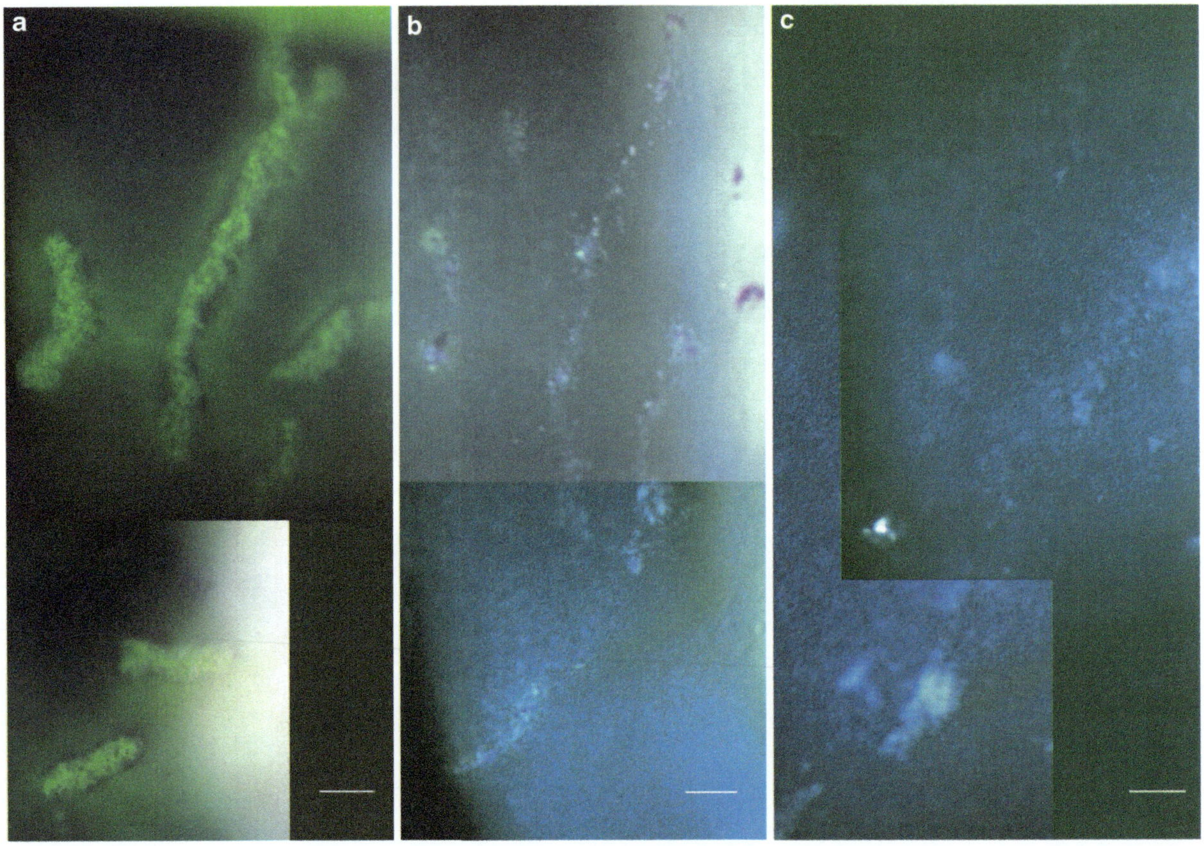

Fig. 3.8 a–c Survey of HSV epithelial lesions before and during treatment with acyclovir ointment. (**a**) Before treatment, the epithelium shows several variously long lesions containing swollen cells. (**b**) After 4 days of treatment with acyclovir ointment, the lesions have diminished in size; the distribution pattern is still recognizable. (**c**) The appearance after 11 days of treatment (composed photographs; for details, see Figs. 3.9 and 3.10 opposite page and Fig. 3.11 overleaf)

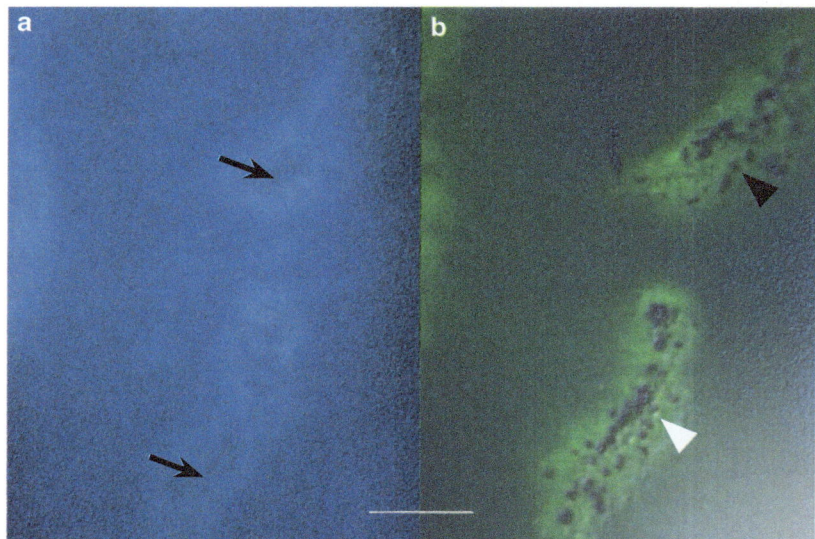

Fig. 3.9 a–b *Before treatment.* (**a**) Before staining, the central parts (*arrows*) of these two lesions appear dark and the surrounding diseased surface epithelium grayish. (**b**) The lesions show swollen/rounded cells (*white arrowhead*). The green staining with fluorescein sodium indicates surface disruptions. Some damaged surface cells stain red with rose bengal (*black arrowhead*)

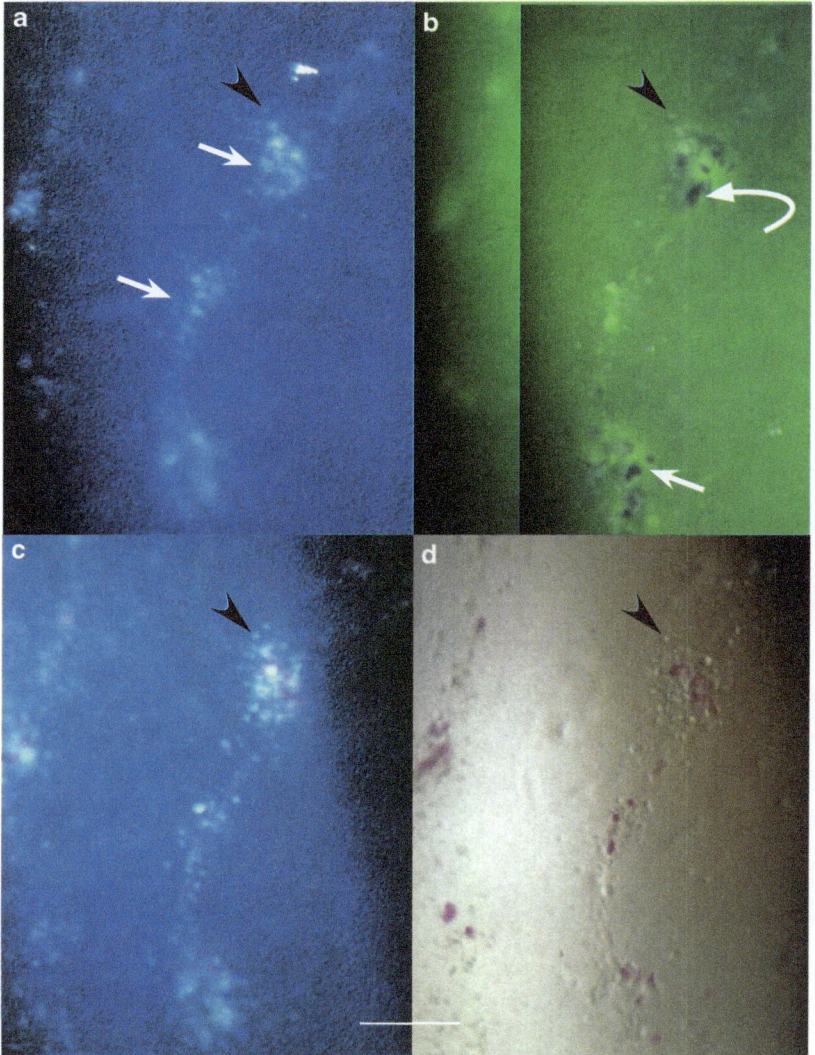

Fig. 3.10 a–d *After 4 days of treatment* with acyclovir ointment, the same area shows the following: (**a**) before staining, individual (*arrowhead*) or grouped (*arrows*) light-reflecting dots; (**b**) with fluorescein sodium, pooling of green-stained tear fluid in some areas (*short arrow*) between protruding (dark) structures (*bowed arrow*); (**c**) an absence of fluorescein diffusion into the tissues; and (**d**) abnormal cells (*arrowhead*) and red rose bengal staining of a few diseased/damaged surface cells/cell debris (the arrowheads are placed in corresponding locations; **b**, composed photograph)

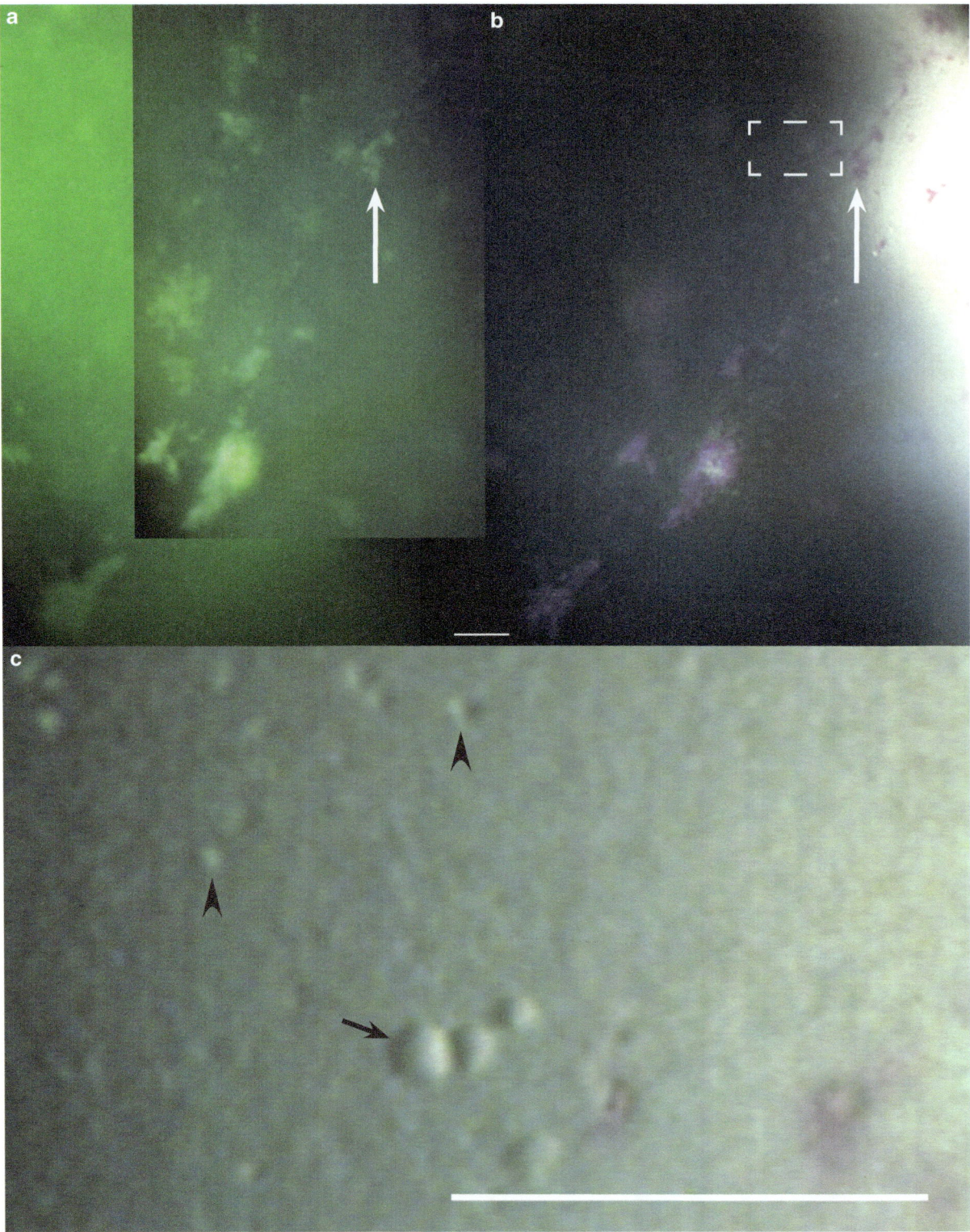

Fig. 3.11 a–c *After 11 days of treatment*, the epithelium shows damaged surface cells; in (**a**) these are visible as bright green dots; the same cells (**b**) stain red with rose bengal (long arrows, placed in corresponding locations). In *frame*, the area shown in (**c**). (**c**) Abnormal cells (*arrowheads*) and small cysts (*black arrow*) (**a**, composed photograph)

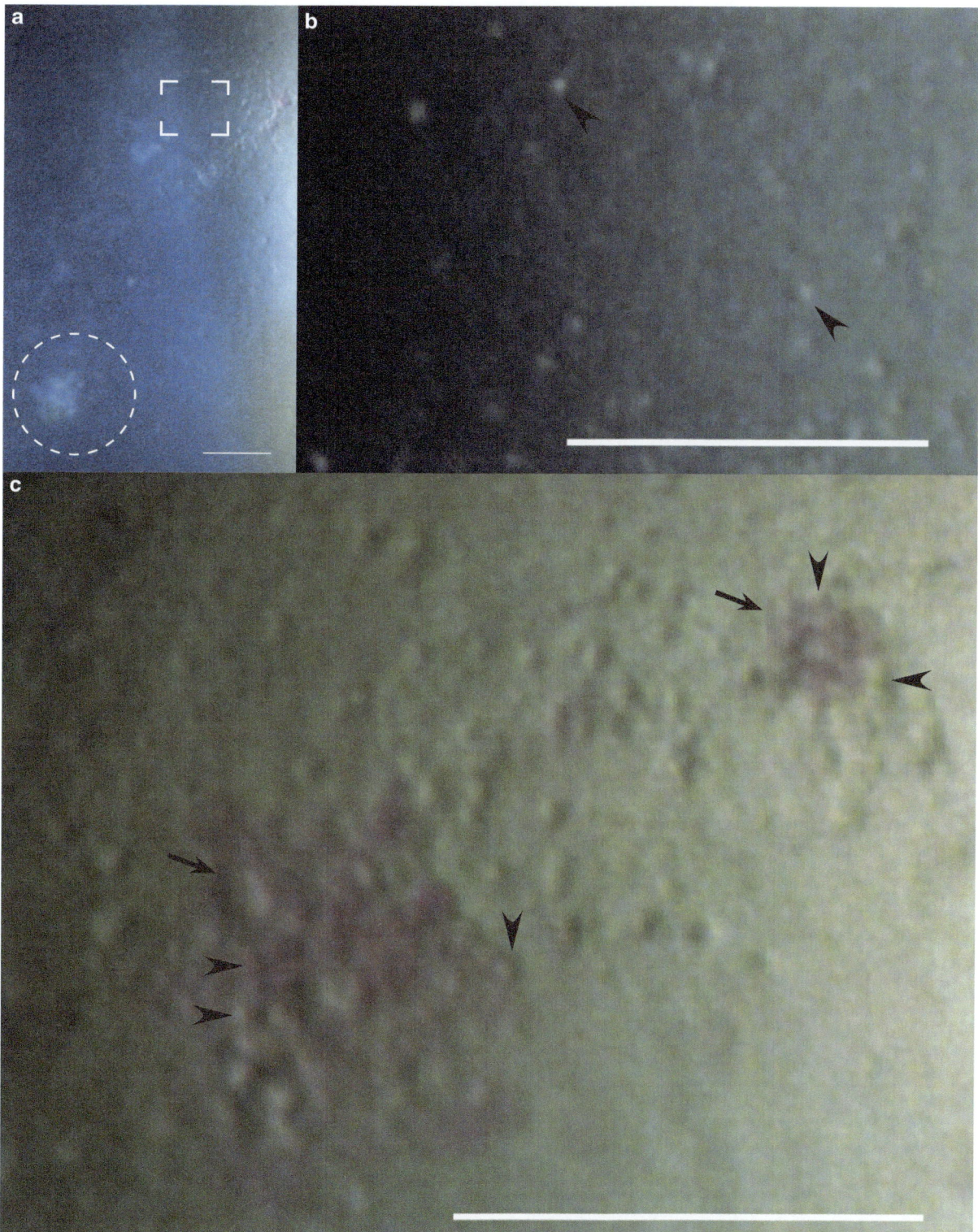

Fig. 3.12 a–c *After 2 weeks of treatment,* the following are visible: (**a**) grayish epithelial patches with the *frames* indicating areas shown at higher magnification level in (**b**) and (**c**); (**b**) rectangular frame shows individual abnormal cells (*arrowheads*); (**c**) circular frame shows rose bengal staining of cell debris (*arrows*) overlying grouped abnormal cells (*arrowheads*)

Healing of HSV Epithelial Keratitis, Accompanying Signs, and Sequelae (Case 2, cont.)

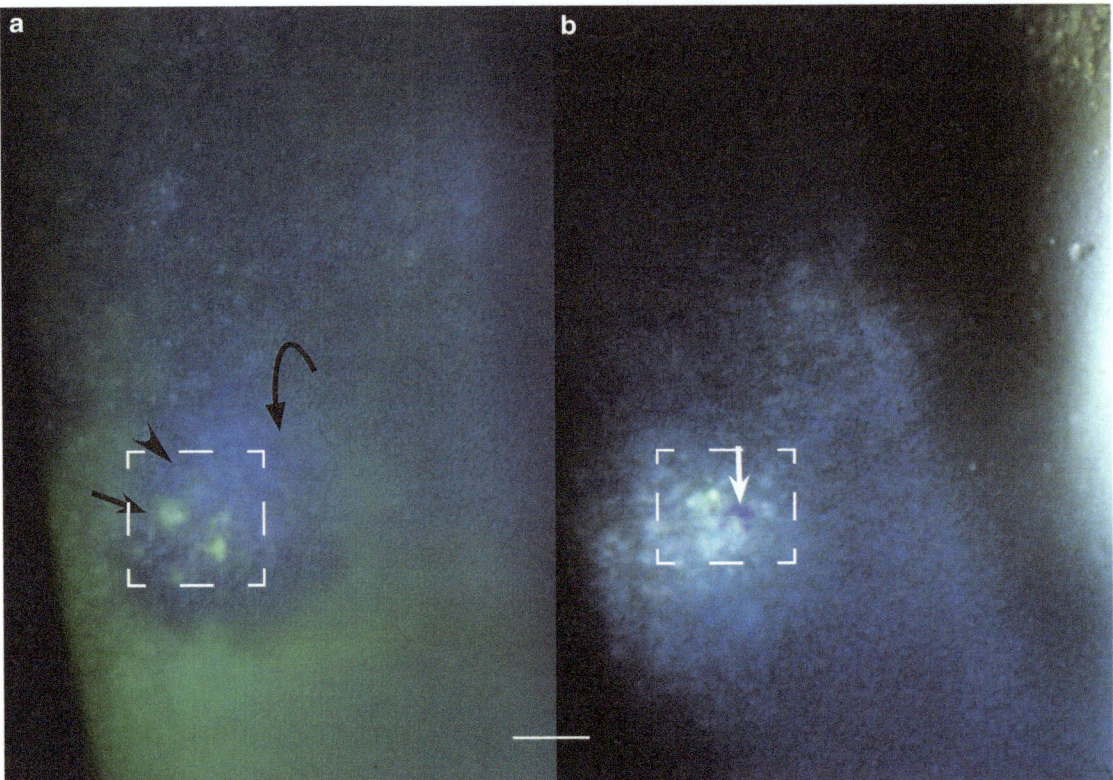

Fig. 3.13 a–b At 4.5 *weeks after onset* of symptoms, the surface shows (**a**) surface elevations (*bowed arrow*) containing bright dots (*arrowhead*) and small cystic spaces (*short black arrow*). The area in *frame* is shown in Fig. 3.14a and b). In (**b**) are visible many bright dots and minimal rose bengal staining (*arrow*) (the area in frame is shown in Fig. 3.15a and b). (The area captured in **a** appears similar to, but is not identical with that in **b**)

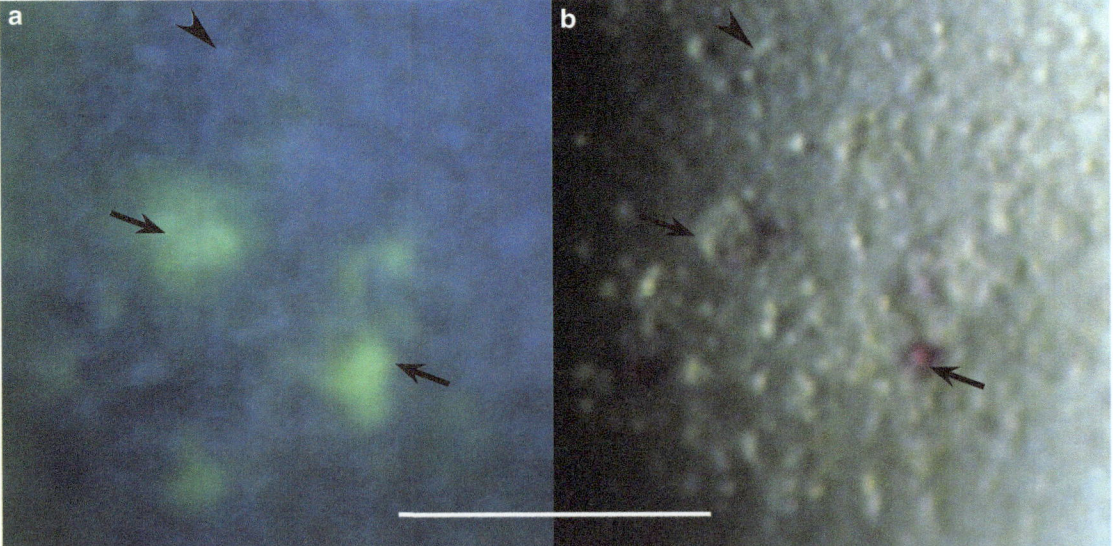

Fig. 3.14 a–b The lower part of Fig. 3.13a shows (**a**) small cystic spaces staining green with fluorescein sodium (*black arrows*) and many grayish dots that are partly confluent (*arrowhead*). (**b**) The area contains many abnormal cells (*arrowhead*), individual or grouped. Diseased surface cells/cell debris stain red with rose bengal (*black arrows*) (the markers are placed in corresponding locations)

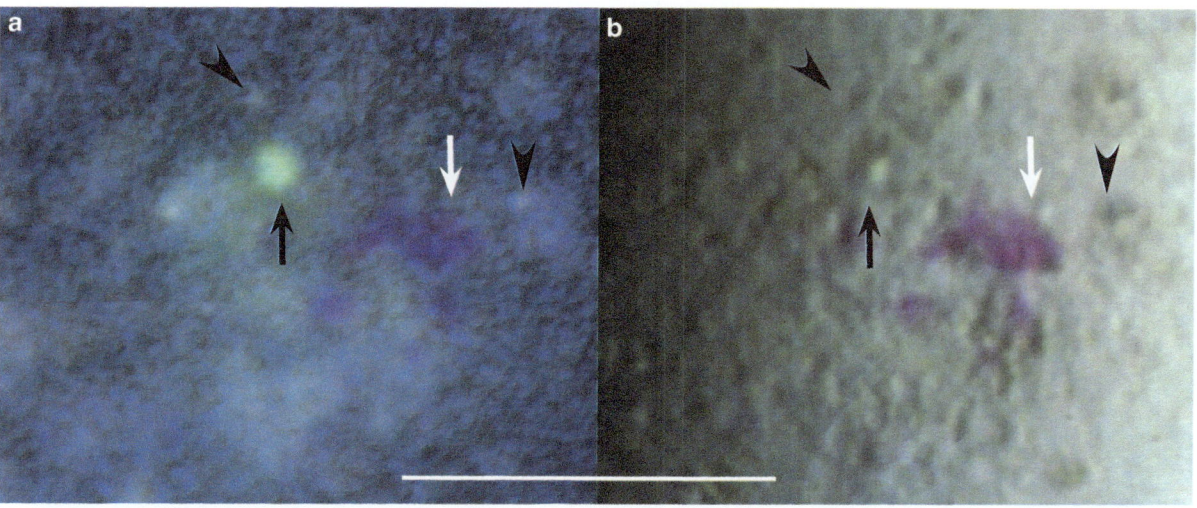

Fig. 3.15 a–b Lower part of the area shown in Fig. 3.13b. (a) Gray dots (*arrowheads*) correspond to (b) abnormal cells (*arrowheads*). There is a small rounded cystic space staining green (*black arrow*); some damaged surface cells/cell debris stain red with rose bengal (*white arrow*) (the markers are placed in corresponding locations)

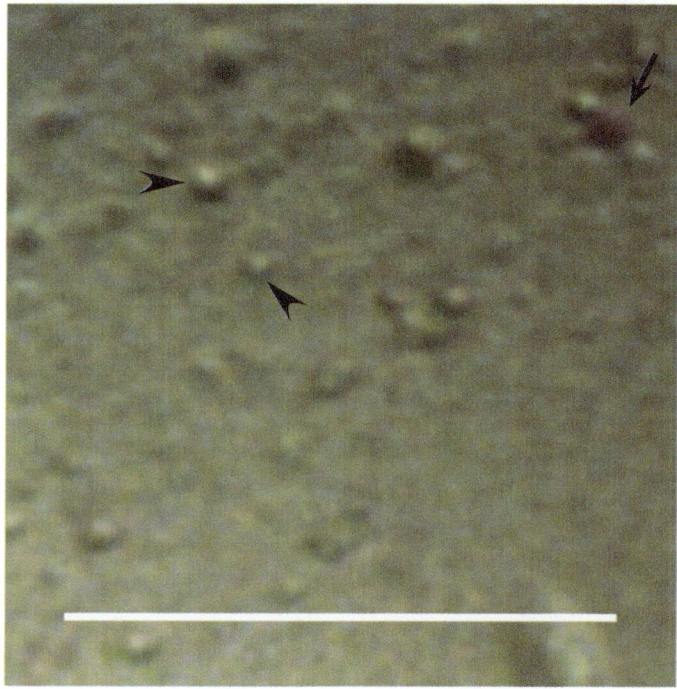

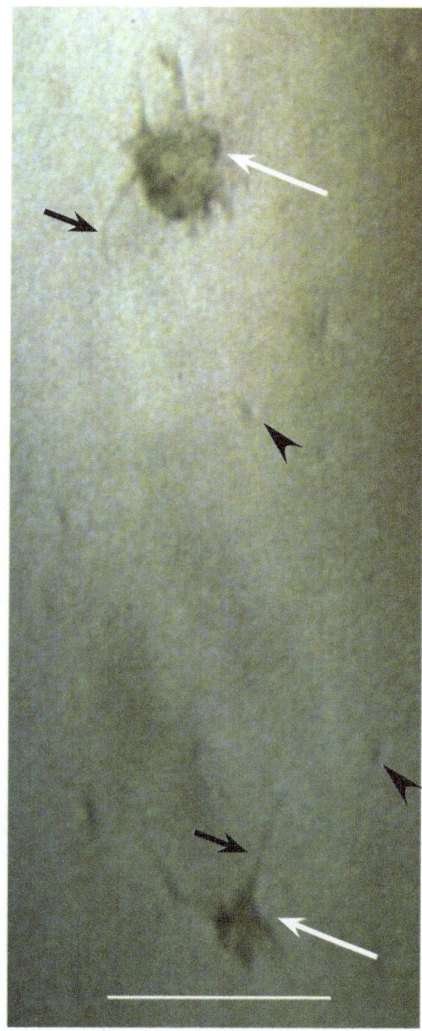

Fig. 3.16 Close view of abnormal cells (*arrowheads*). The *arrow* indicates a damaged surface cell staining with rose bengal

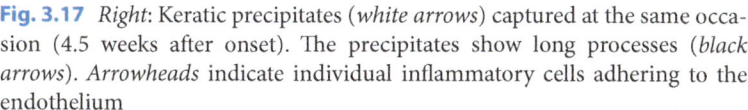

Fig. 3.17 *Right*: Keratic precipitates (*white arrows*) captured at the same occasion (4.5 weeks after onset). The precipitates show long processes (*black arrows*). *Arrowheads* indicate individual inflammatory cells adhering to the endothelium

Healing of HSV Epithelial Keratitis, Accompanying Signs, and Sequelae (Case 2, cont.)

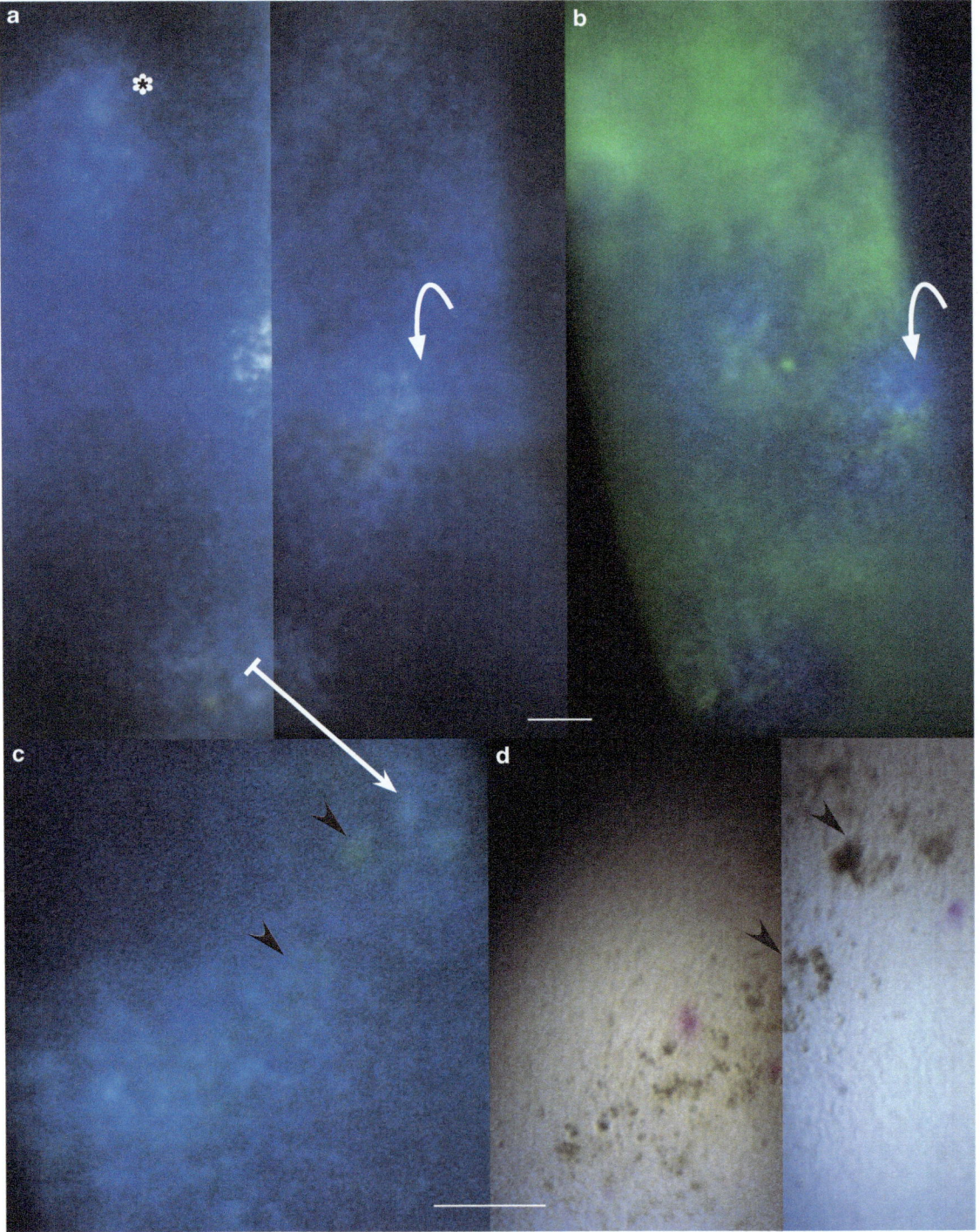

Fig. 3.18 a–d *Nine weeks after onset,* the following are visible: (**a**) grayish opacities (*bowed arrow*) that are (**b**) partly elevated (dark; *bowed arrow*) (the asterisk indicates a reference point for comparison with Fig. 3.19; the *long arrow* indicates the location of the area shown at higher magnification in **c** and **d**); (**c**) the patterns of the light-reflecting structures within the opacities (*arrowheads*) corresponding to those of (**d**) abnormal cells, clustered or individual (*arrowheads*). (The arrows/arrowheads are placed in corresponding locations; **a** and **d** are composed photographs)

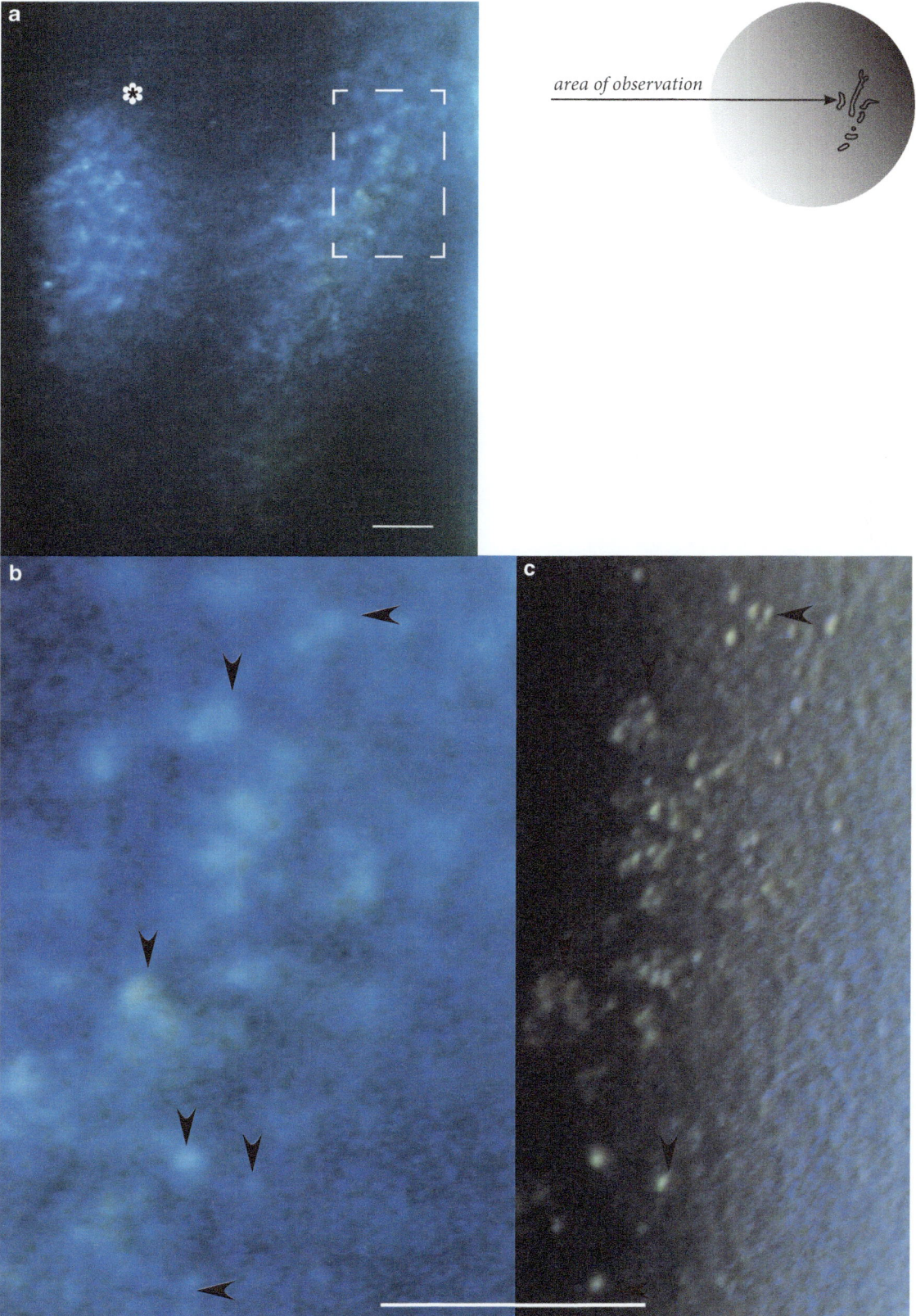

Fig. 3.19 a–c The appearance *10 months after onset of symptoms* of the grayish (light-reflecting) opacities. (**a**) The asterisk indicates the same area as in Fig. 3.18a (cf. also drawing). The area in frame is shown in (**b**) and (**c**). (**b, c**) The light-reflecting dots (**b**) correspond to grouped or individual abnormal cells (**c**). (The arrowheads are placed in corresponding locations)

Healing of HSV Epithelial Keratitis, Accompanying Signs, and Sequelae (Case 2, cont.)

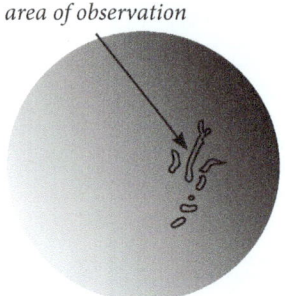

area of observation

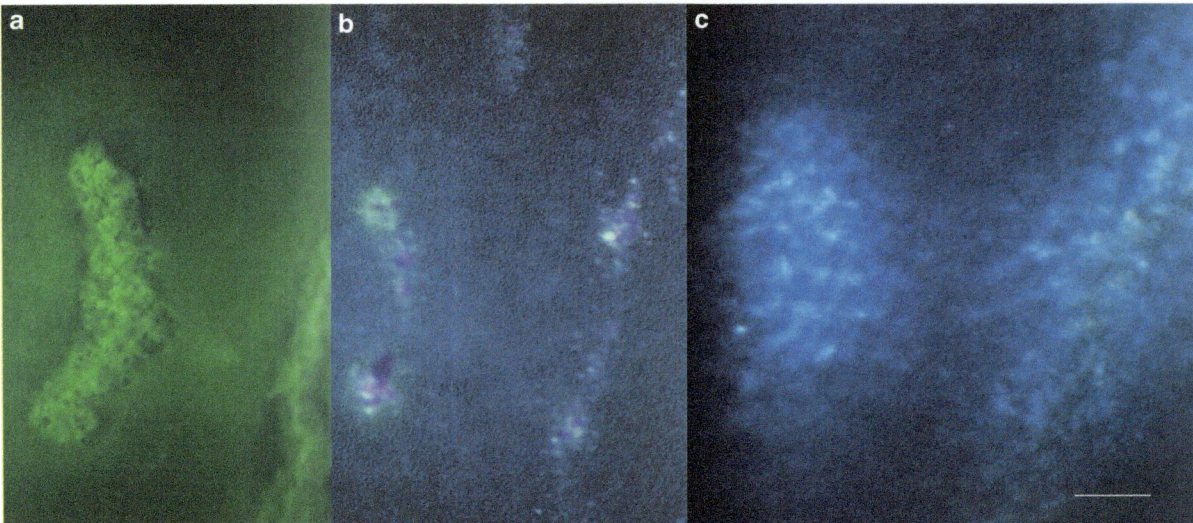

Fig. 3.20 a–c Survey of development in the area indicated in the drawing (above). (**a**) Epithelial changes caused by *HSV infection*, captured after 7 days of symptoms. (**b**) The appearance *after 4 days of treatment* with acyclovir ointment five times a day. (**c**) Subepithelial opacities present *10 months after onset* of symptoms

Addendum

Six years after the episode described here, stromal infiltrates developed at 11 and 1 o'clock close to the corneal limbus. Two months later, disciform keratitis located centroparacentrally in the nasal part of the cornea appeared. Later, after 7 years symptom free, the patient suffered two recurrences of stromal keratitis at the superior limbus. After 17 years, the area shown in Fig. 3.20 was still well discernible with the slit lamp as a superficial grayish shadow.

Case 3. HSV Epithelial Keratitis and Stromal Infiltrates

Case Report

Six years before these photographs were taken, this 45-year-old woman with no history of eye disease presented with redness, irritation, photophobia, and pain in the right eye. The symptoms started 3 days previously. The cornea showed two whitish and partly ulcerated infiltrates at 8 and 11 o'clock, close to the limbus. She was treated with topical antibiotics and cortisone. The infiltrates resolved within 8 days.

Six years later, the right eye became inflamed again. At presentation, the duration of symptoms was 10 days. The cornea showed two whitish infiltrates located at 5 and 11 o'clock close to the limbus, accompanied by a small HSV-suspect epithelial lesion. On questioning, the patient reported that she had been suffering from blisters in her mouth for many years, and that the latest attack had occurred 2 weeks previously. She was treated with acyclovir ointment five times a day. Five days later, all signs of active epithelial infection were gone, and the infiltrates were smaller. After a further week of treatment, all inflammatory signs were gone. Virus isolation test in cell culture revealed HSV type 1 (HSV-1).

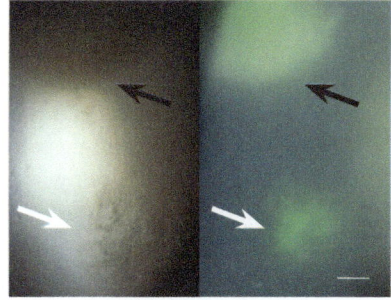

Fig. 3.21 *Left*: An *infiltrate* (*black arrow*) and an *epithelial lesion* (*white arrow*). *Right*: Both partly stain green with fluorescein sodium

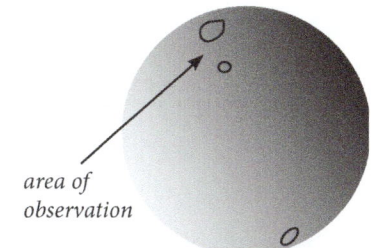

area of observation

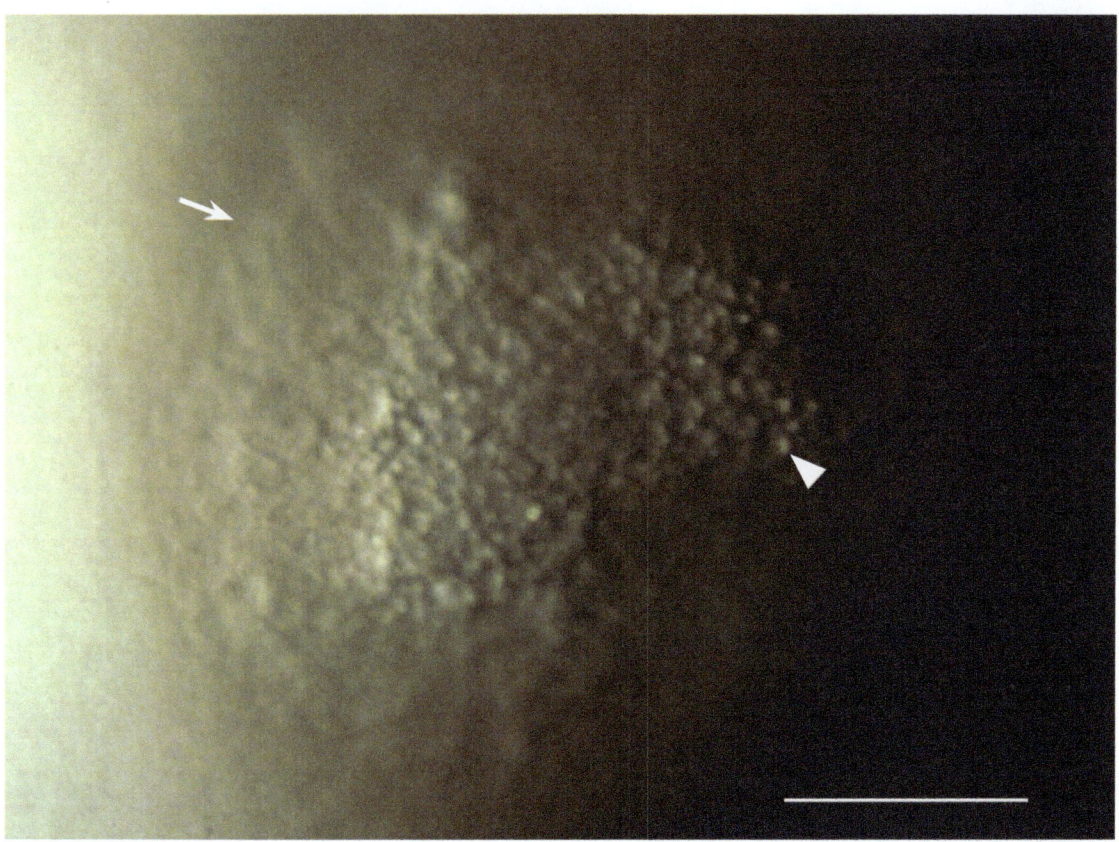

Fig. 3.22 HSV epithelial lesion (*arrow*) located close to a stromal infiltrate (Fig. 3.21). The lesion shows many swollen/rounded cells (*arrowhead*)

Case 4. HSV Epithelial Keratitis Preceded by Anterior Uveitis and Disciform Keratitis

Case Report

A 50-year-old man was diagnosed with left-sided anterior uveitis and treated with topical steroids and cycloplegics. A month after the treatment was stopped, he presented again, this time with a disciform keratitis, keratic precipitates, and a mild anterior uveitis. HSV origin was suspected. Four months after onset of the first symptoms, the lower part of the cornea showed three small HSV-suspect epithelial lesions. At that occasion, HSV-1 infection was verified in cell culture.

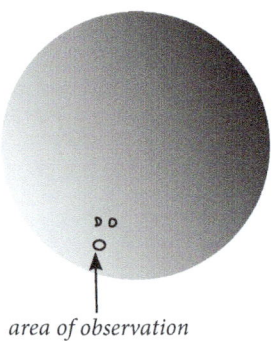

area of observation

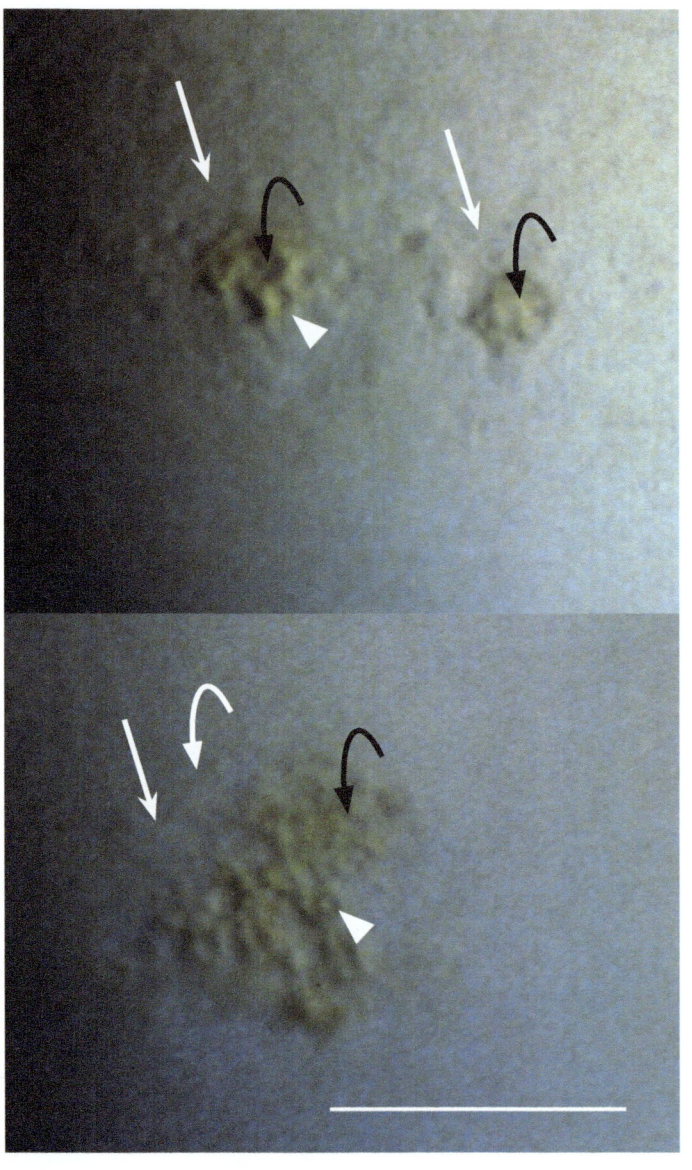

Fig. 3.23 Three small HSV epithelial lesions (*straight arrows*). The lesions show swollen/rounded cells (*arrowhead*) and central depressions (*black bowed arrows*) in which fluorescein-stained tear fluid is pooling (appearing slightly yellow in this illumination). The periphery of the lesions seems elevated (*white bowed arrow*) (composed photograph)

The epithelial keratitis healed with acyclovir ointment. After that, the cornea showed a mild disciform keratitis, which was treated with low-dose steroids. All attempts to stop the steroids, however slowly tapered, resulted in a recurrence of the keratitis accompanied by anterior uveitis. During this period, dry eye was diagnosed. Four years after onset of the first symptoms of an HSV-related inflammation, while on 0.1% prednisolone sodium phosphate eye drops every other day, the left eye again became irritated. The patient started to use the steroid drops more frequently. After 2 weeks, the cornea showed a large dendritic figure (Figs. 3.24 and 3.25).

Addendum

The epithelial keratitis healed with acyclovir ointment five times a day. During the following 11 years, disciform keratitis waxed and waned. There were no further episodes of epithelial keratitis.

HSV Epithelial Keratitis and Dry Eye (Case 4, cont.)

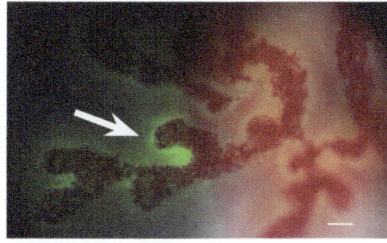

Fig. 3.24 A part of a large HSV epithelial lesion. Close view of the area indicated by *arrow* is shown in Fig. 3.25

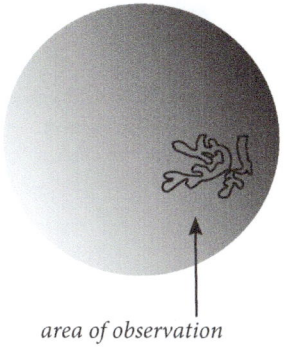

area of observation

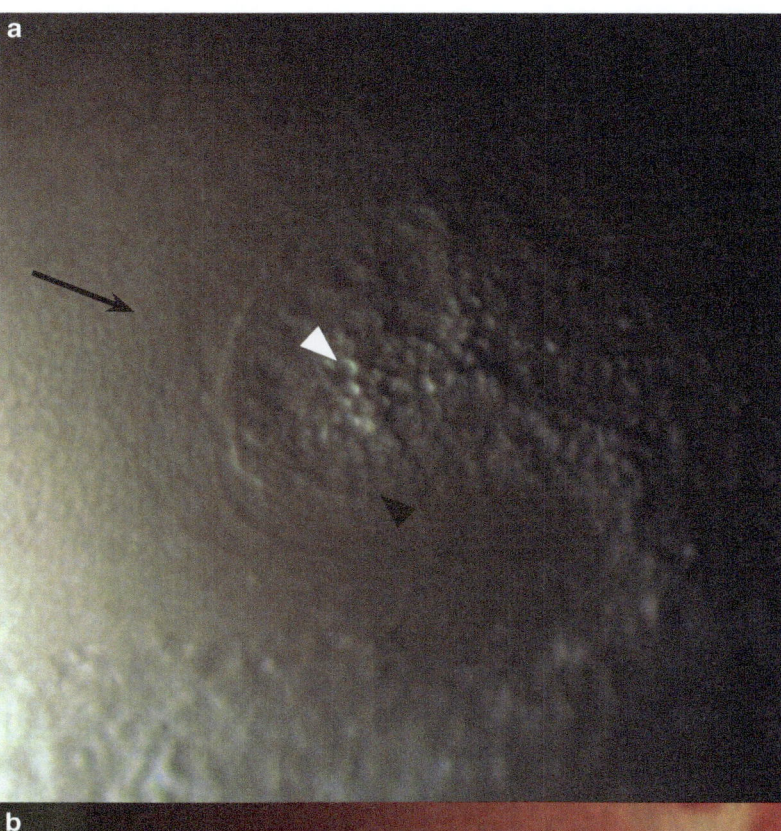

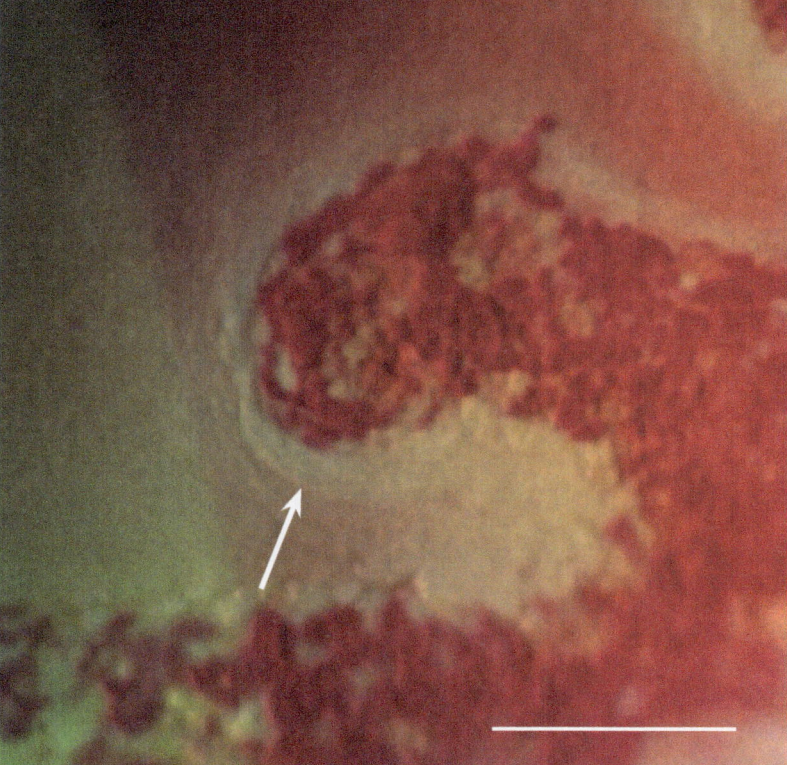

Fig. 3.25 a–b (**a**) The lesion shows many "bright" (*white arrowhead*) and "dull" (*black arrowhead*) swollen/rounded cells. Visible in the surroundings is fine (basal) epithelial edema (*arrow*). (**b**) Diseased surface cells/cell debris within the same part of the lesion stain heavily with rose bengal. The surrounding bright halo (*arrow*) is caused by fluorescein diffusion (cf. Fig. 3.24). The tear fluid is concurrently stained red with rose bengal dye

Case 5. Recurrent HSV Epithelial Keratitis in a Patient with Dry Eye

Case Report

In a healthy 71-year-old woman, the first known attack of HSV dendritic keratitis in her left eye occurred in the lower temporal cornea. Four years later, the lower part of the cornea developed disciform keratitis. After that, she was also diagnosed with dry eye. During the following 9 years, she suffered several relapses of stromal keratitis and mild or severe anterior uveitis and seven recurrences of epithelial keratitis occurring in the temporal, nasal, or central cornea. With time, she developed a large and dense stromal opacity involving almost the whole cornea. Nineteen years after the first attack, a small area of corneal melting was successfully treated with glue and a contact lens.

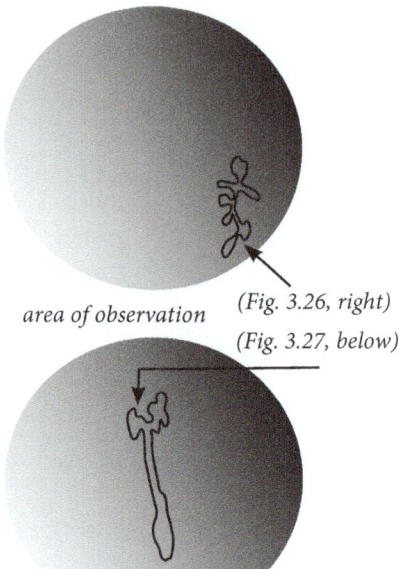

area of observation   (Fig. 3.26, right)
    (Fig. 3.27, below)

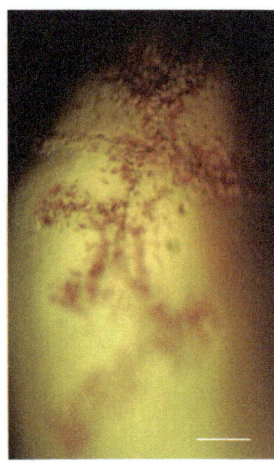

Fig. 3.26 A large dendritic figure in the lower temporal part of the cornea

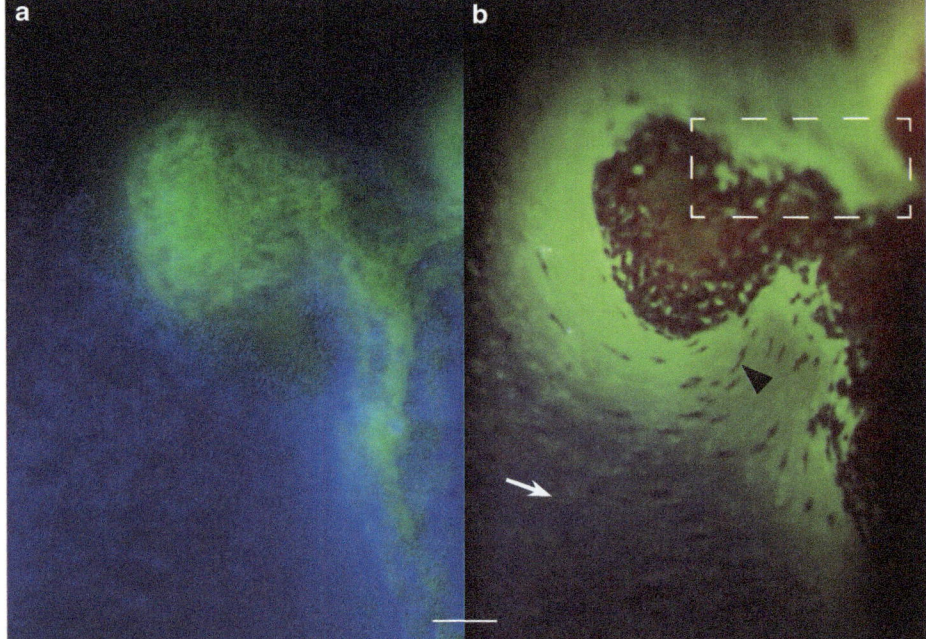

Fig. 3.27 a–b The left upper part of a large dendritic HSV lesion running vertically from 12 to 6 o'clock over the central cornea (cf. drawing). Sixth recurrence, 13 years after the first known HSV epithelial infection. (**a**) The lesion, captured shortly after application of fluorescein sodium, stains vividly, but there is no diffusion into the surroundings yet. No green punctate staining in the surrounding epithelium is visible. (**b**) After a minute or two, there is extensive fluorescein diffusion into the surroundings. The lesion stains heavily with rose bengal. The surroundings show rose bengal-stained cells (*arrowhead*) and green dots (*arrow*); the area within the *frame* is shown in Fig. 3.28

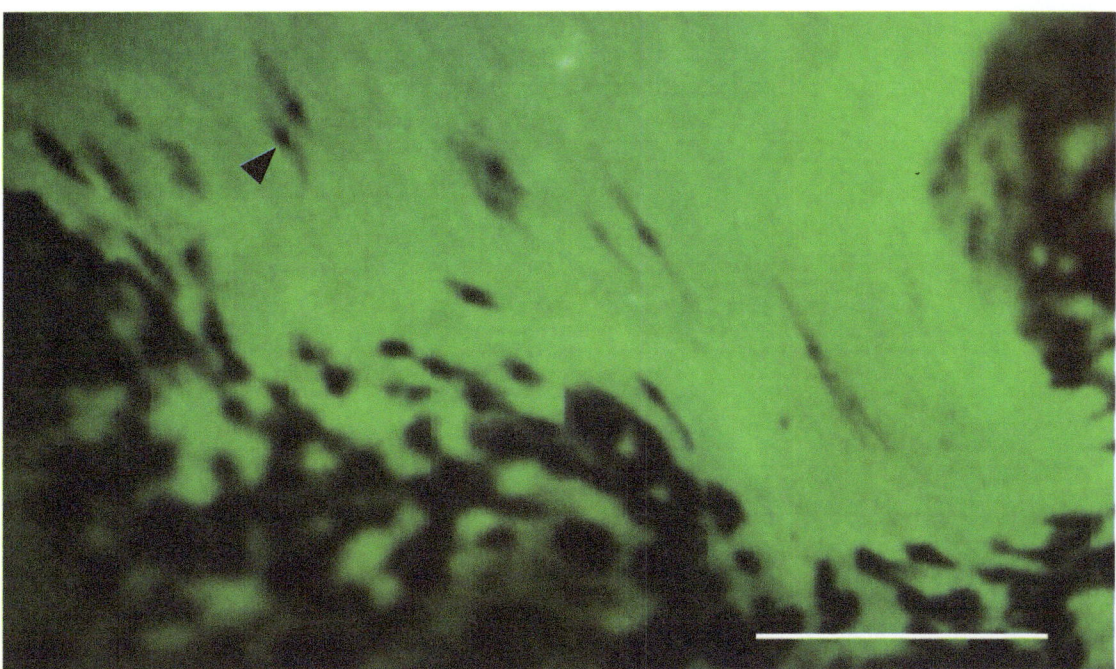

Fig. 3.28 Close view of the area indicated by frame in Fig. 3.27. Some rose bengal-stained superficial cells outside the dendritic figure appear fusiform and show densely stained nuclei (*arrowhead*)

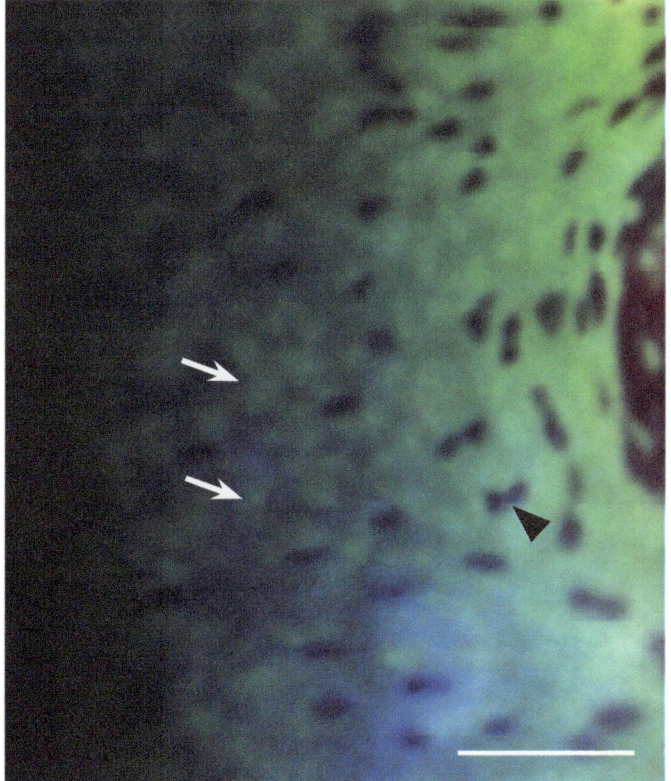

Fig. 3.29 In addition to rose bengal-stained cells (*arrowhead*), the epithelium outside the dendritic figure shows green dots (*arrows*) caused by toxic effect of rose bengal

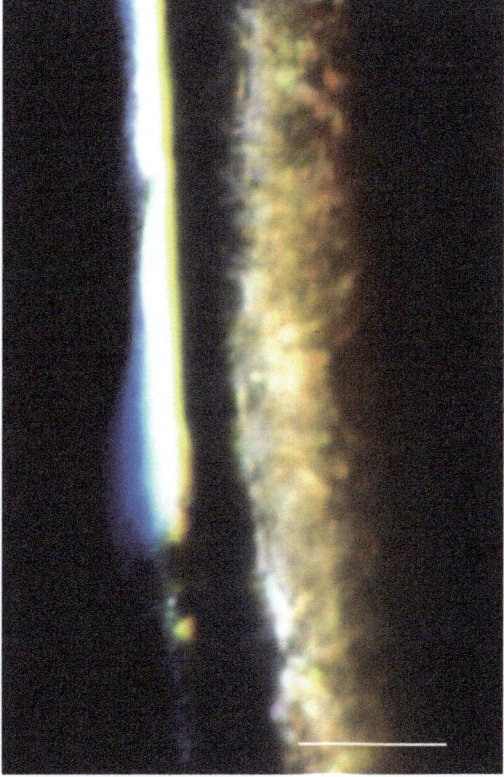

Fig. 3.30 This stromal scarring, captured 14 years after the first occasion of HSV epithelial keratitis shown in Fig. 3.26, is not a sequela of epithelial but of stromal keratitis

Bibliography

1. Tabery HM (1992) Dual appearance of fluorescein staining in vivo of diseased human corneal epithelium. A non-contact photomicrographic study. Br J Ophthalmol 76:43–44
2. Tabery HM (1995) Morphology of herpes simplex dendritic keratitis. A non-contact photomicrographic study in vivo in the human cornea. Herpes 2:55–57
3. Tabery HM (1997) Micropunctate staining of the human corneal surface: micro-erosions or cystic spaces? A non-contact photomicrographic in vivo study. Acta Ophthalmol Scand 75:134-136
4. Tabery HM (1998) Toxic effect of rose bengal dye on the living human corneal epithelium. Acta Ophthalmol Scand 7:142–145
5. Tabery HM (1998) Early epithelial changes in recurrent herpes simplex virus keratitis. A non-contact photomicrographic study in vivo in the human cornea. Acta Ophthalmol Scand 76:349–352
6. Tabery HM (2000) Epithelial changes in early primary herpes simplex virus keratitis. Photomicrographic observations in a case of human infection. Acta Opthalmol Scand 78:706–709
7. Tabery HM (2001) Healing of recurrent herpes simplex corneal epithelial lesions treated with topical acyclovir. A non-contact photomicrographic in vivo study in the human cornea. Acta Ophthalmol Scand 79:256–261
8. Tabery HM (2003) Corneal surface changes in keratoconjunctivitis sicca. Part I: the surface proper. A non-contact photomicrographic in vivo study in the human cornea. Eye 17:482–487
9. Tabery HM, Holm O (1987) Photography in vivo of epithelial lesions in the human cornea. Acta Ophthalmol (Copenh) 65:513–514

Index